Unknown Warrior

BATTLING *the* MIRROR

For you, by Sar

SARAH CALLAZZO

Copyright © 2024 Sarah Callazzo.

All rights reserved.

No part of this publication may be reproduced, distributed or transmitted in any form or by any means, including photocopying, recording or other electronic or mechanical methods, without the prior written permission of the publisher, except in the case of brief quotations, reviews and other noncommercial uses permitted by copyright law.

Katie
Mom and Dad
My family
My friends who became family
Erica, Jenny, Karen
and My Angels,

I owe everything to you.

To younger Sar and every single person who has been a part of my journey: this one's for you.

"You know, sometimes all you need is twenty seconds of insane courage. Just literally twenty seconds of embarrassing bravery. And I promise you, something great will come of it."
—Benjamin Mee, *We Bought a Zoo*

This quote led me to recovery, this book, and ultimately all of you. My health, my 20 seconds tattoo, and my published words mean more to me than I will ever be able to express.

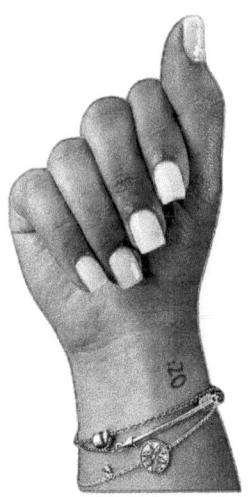

Throughout our time together, I hope you:

Fold pages that resonate with you and share them with those who need them most.
Find the strength to talk about your struggles and inspire others to do the same.

I hope you laugh.
I hope you tear up in the most beautiful way.
I hope you feel safe, seen, and supported.

I hope you recognize your pain and realize how strong you are to have made it through the things you never thought you could.

If this book gets one conversation started . . .
If one page has the words you didn't know you needed to hear . . .
If one line helps you look at just one day a little differently . . .
then every ounce of my heartache was worth it.

I didn't know it at the time, but I've been subconsciously writing this book for years.
I hope you enjoy it.
xo

Before the beginning . . .

BEFORE THE BEGINNING . . .

When it comes to learning to love your body, I may not have all the answers, but I am someone who has been there.

Whether you are actively fighting your thoughts, struggling to keep them inside, or pretending everything is okay, I hear you.

And guess what? I'm proud of you. I'm so unbelievably proud of you for making it to today.

If you are hurting, learning to live in a different body, facing your Goliath, or celebrating your wins . . . I see you. I am rooting for you and I am inspired by you for every single step you have taken and will take on this journey.

*The information provided within these pages is based on my personal journey and life experiences. By participating in reading my words, you acknowledge that I am not a licensed psychologist, medical doctor, or healthcare professional, and my services do not replace the care from them.

Author's note

My initial plan was to organize this book into chapters titled "The Sunrise," "The Storm," "The Sunset," and "Somewhere around 2 a.m."

I read each page and tried to decide which "time of day" it fit into. It was at that moment I learned more about my recovery than I did in five years of being in it. Each page was written about a day of my journey, and looking back on it, it is almost impossible to say if it was blissful or disastrous in its entirety. The memory embodies both, and everything in between.

So, I present to you my rollercoaster of a recovery. It is a beautiful mess. There were some days I could've sworn I was chained to rock bottom. There were other days I felt like I could fly.

But I guess if I wasn't ebbing and flowing, I wouldn't have been healing.

BEFORE THE BEGINNING . . .

Katie may be younger than I, but she will always be the person I look up to.

She is my pride and joy: the best thing that has ever happened to me.
She leaves everywhere she goes better than she found it.
She has the brightest light radiating inside of her.
She is kind, hysterical, talented, and selfless.
She is unbelievably beautiful.

Every argument only lasts a few minutes and normally ends with a McDonald's cookie tote.
Every car ride turns into our own private concert and dance party.
Every moment with her is one that I cherish most.

She taught me what it means to live.
She taught me what it means to be a big sister.
She truly has given me the greatest honor of all.

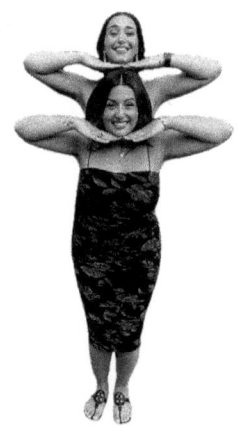

I love you more than you love doing puzzles, bbyk8.

Growing up, my mom told me "Greatest Love of All" by Whitney Houston was one of her favorite songs. I never understood why, because, at the time, the Jonas Brothers sang my favorite song.

Now that I am twenty-five, I've realized that not only was my mom always right, but she knew me better than I knew myself all along.

My mom taught me how to be strong.
She is the type of person who epitomizes all that is good in the world.
She never takes anything for granted and she pays everything she has forward.
She has the very best heart.
She was put on this earth to be a mother, and I am so lucky she is mine.

For me, "Greatest Love of All" will always be a song that feels like home.

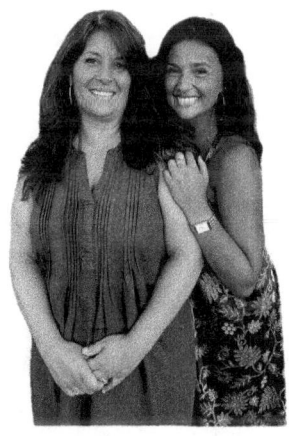

I love you, Mom.

BEFORE THE BEGINNING . . .

I grew up a competitive dancer and I thought my dad didn't understand my competitions.

He always said awards are given because of three people's opinions at one point in time.
I didn't care to listen to him because, at that moment, those three opinions meant everything to me.

Looking back on it, I guess he was onto something, and I wish I was able to hear his words more clearly.

He wasn't saying "You should've won." He was saying, "You shouldn't take their critiques further than an evaluation of how you performed. You should not base your worth on others' opinions. You shouldn't try to dance or be like anyone else but you. You should never underestimate yourself."

I don't think he ever thought he'd be a girl dad, but he is the greatest one of all.

Dad, you are the best mentor, wine-drinking buddy, and other half of the dynamic duo a girl could ask for.

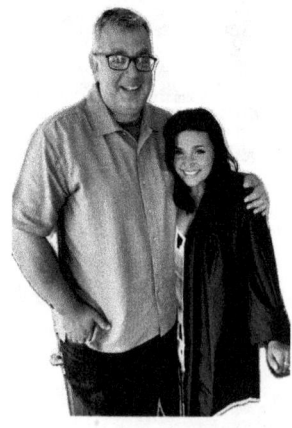

I'll always be your "baby chicken." I love you, worldwide.

I've lived in so many bodies, all of which I never thought were "good enough." For years, I tried to fill an anxiety-ridden void with eating disorder behaviors. In doing so, I found out the hard way that it wouldn't bring me the overwhelming joy I was looking for. I tried everything I could to "fix" my body, only to realize it was never the problem to begin with.

I have always been worthy of acceptance, respect, and love, even though I had a hard time believing it. I never thought my body was worthy of being on the cover of a book . . . and yet here I am.

My artist, Heather, painted my form in a way which allowed me to be free of my thoughts that used to be all-consuming. She allowed me to celebrate the vessel that has carried me through life, even though it is a little bit bigger than it used to be. I have gained necessary weight during eating disorder recovery. But the strength, respect, and love I have gained for myself in the process has been worth every pound.

My photographer, Ruben, began the photoshoot by asking me what I felt when I was struggling most: Broken. Lost. Unworthy. Defeated. I had tears in my eyes while trying to explain my feelings to him because this was one of the first times I voiced it out loud. And it was one of the first times I was able to see how far I've truly come.

Thank you, Heather and Ruben, for turning a body I used to be ashamed of into art.

Heather Deegean Hires & Ruben D. Garcia
#bodypaintingbyheather #thephotographyofrubendgarcia

2017
the year of firsts

Sometimes the strongest thing you can do is ask for help. Every other Thursday morning, I talk to a therapist and a certified eating disorder dietician. This dedicated team of professionals has become my lifeline, offering guidance and support that has changed my life in ways I never imagined.

If you are looking for a sign from the universe that now is the time to make an appointment, this page is it.

https://www.edreferral.com/easysearch

https://www.psychologytoday.com/us

I freaking love therapy . . .

2017

. . . But I didn't always.

I often look back and laugh about my first therapy session. I was twelve years old, and let's just say my therapist and I were less than a perfect match.

She offered me a chicken nugget from a box that was sitting on the floor beside her dog.
She said that if I needed a tissue, I could take one from the tiki's nose hanging on her wall.
She said to never watch *Jersey Shore* and continued to lecture me on that topic for around a half hour. (I had never seen the show and wasn't planning on starting it anytime soon.)

It was a disaster and I swore I was never going back to therapy.
Five years later, I did, and to this day, it is the best decision I have ever made.

Don't get discouraged.
Keep searching until you find the person who will change your life.
They are out there, I promise.

There is no such thing as a universal truth in human perception. This means, when it comes to preference or opinion, there isn't a single standard that can be applied to an entire population.

Let's break it down. Do you have a favorite pizza topping? Is there anything anyone could say to make your opinion waver? Even if every person in the world agreed and told you better toppings existed, no one could convince you otherwise, right?

You could ask one hundred different people what their favorite topping is, and you could potentially have one hundred different answers: pepperoni, mushroom, pineapple (hehe), etc. . . .

That's a really beautiful thing.
Now imagine if we felt that way about our bodies . . . not as easy, is it?

We are much more impressionable when it comes to our sense of self, and the media knows that. They don't waste their time saying, "pepperoni is the best pizza topping." But they do focus a lot of time and energy into convincing us, "every other body is better than the one you have."

They tried to create a universal truth about beauty . . . and we bought into it.

It seems so silly to try and put a universal truth on something like a pizza topping.
We all know there is no one supreme topping everyone in the world could agree on. So why do we accept it when it comes to our bodies?

Instead of trying to fit into the unattainable standards society has set for us, find yourself and then find your people to share a pizza with.

Yeah, I learned this in therapy.

2017

cel·lu·lite
noun
a cosmetic, localized skin condition that causes a dimpled appearance on the surface of the skin.

For too many individuals, cellulite is defined as weakness, unattractiveness, or failure. But, my dear, an indent on your leg is not worth hating yourself over.

Here is your permission to show off your legs . . . even if your thighs have cute little dimples.
Here is your permission to wear your favorite pair of shorts and light-colored leggings . . . even in the sunlight.
Here is your permission to be kind to yourself. And to love your legs, cellulite and all.

#celluLIT
#thighdimple

I was eighteen when the doctors found a tumor on the sheath of my brain: eosinophilic granuloma. It wasn't a physical tumor, but one that caused my skull to erode. When the doctors went in for surgery, they tapped my skull, and it shattered like an eggshell. I now have a cute little titanium plate in my head replacing the broken piece of my skull.

On the anniversary of my surgery, people always ask me how I am feeling, emotionally. All I can ever come up with is "I am feeling a lot."

I still remember getting wheeled into surgery. I felt a sense of guilt because everything I put such heavy value on suddenly meant nothing. All the accolades, grades, and compliments I worked so hard for were instantly just . . . meaningless.

Want to know what I *wasn't* thinking on my way into surgery?

- *Thank God you restricted yourself the other night and didn't allow yourself to enjoy a meal with your friends!*
- *Congrats, you wear a size 4 now instead of a size 6!*
- *I am so glad you spent more time looking in a mirror than you did looking at the world around you! It was worth it!*

Instead, I thought:

- *At the end of the day, your body did some amazing things, and it's always been beautiful.*
- *Your anxiety doesn't define you.*
- *Enjoy every little moment you have after this because right now you don't know when your next one will be.*

I find myself needing that reminder sometimes. I am so thankful for my doctors, my friends, and my family. It may have taken some time, but I am making the girl getting wheeled into surgery proud, and I can't wait to keep doing it.

July 26 will always be a day I feel grounded.
Seven years tumor-free—forever to go.

I see a new chapter of my life ahead of me.

I see the natural light peeking through my curtains.

I see a stack of books I cannot wait to read.

I see my bedhead reflection in the mirror.

I see greenery and pictures around my room that make this new space feel like home.

I see my passion for art, in all forms, expanding.

I see a beautiful day ahead. A beautiful life ahead.

I cannot wait to get out of my bed and live it.

A "Sunrise" page: what I saw my first morning in Rhode Island.

2017

When was the first time you felt like you weren't good enough?

Journal Prompt 1.0

2018
the year of bliss

2018

I don't really remember the girl I was before 2019.

Throughout 2018, I quickly entered a honeymoon phase of eating disorder recovery where I was fueling my body. I was a little bit bigger, but definitely stronger and happier.

I made my college dance team, got elected president of my sorority, had a boyfriend, and accomplished a 3.96 GPA. I thought I was experiencing freedom around food. I wasn't homesick. I was making friends. Everything was just so good.

2019
the year I found out rock bottom had a basement

Maybe my eating is a little bit disordered, but everyone goes on diets. I'm sure this is normal.

No one around me seems concerned so I definitely don't need therapy or treatment.

I am not thin enough to have anorexia and I only purge when I am consuming alcohol so I don't have bulimia. I don't fit into a "category" so I guess I'm okay.

Ever felt like this before? I promise, you aren't the only one.

For years, I convinced myself I had everything under control. Only recently have I been able to look back and see how severe my negative body image and disordered eating was. Now, living in a bigger (and healthier) body, it's even harder to accept help because I've been taught "people of my size don't have eating disorders."

So please, forget everything you've heard. Eating disorders look different on everyone. There is a large spectrum of severity, and the media only portrays a small piece of it.

There is no such thing as "sick enough."

You deserve more than this.
You deserve help.
You deserve to live a life you love in a body you love.

#BreaktheStigma

I was going to stay private.
I was going to keep this to myself.
I was going to fight this battle on my own.

I normally don't mind being vulnerable. I shake the nerves by hoping my journey will resonate with someone else's. But, for whatever reason, this one was much harder.

I slowly started to open up and the more people I confided in, the more people I realized were going through something so similar. They just needed someone to say it first...

And then it hit me. The only reason I didn't want to talk about this was because no one else was.

So, here I am. Starting the much-needed conversation about normalizing prescribed medication.

If you want the long, sappy page detailing how I got from point A to point B, I'll be more than happy to write it. But, for now, I'm going to leave it at this:

If you had a physical illness, a broken bone, or just weren't feeling well, you wouldn't think twice about seeking help. Whether that be making a doctor's appointment or taking a prescribed antibiotic, you would do whatever it took to feel better.

So why is anxiety medication seen as any different? Why the hell is it so damn hard to do this when it comes to your mental health?

All I want to say is it's okay.

2019

It's okay to need medication, whether it's temporary or long term. It's okay to need therapy, *because how beautiful is it that someone dedicated their life's work to help people just like you?*

It's okay to need a little extra support sometimes—we all do.

It's okay, my love. It's okay.

You are not alone and you deserve to heal.

Every time I'm on a plane and it reaches its altitude, I take a moment to say hi to my angel up there. My girl up there. My hero up there.

I've looked up to her since the moment we met.
I've missed her immeasurably since the moment we parted.
And I will do everything I can to make her proud until the moment we meet again.

Maybe that's why I love flying so much, Dom, because it makes me feel closer to you.

To know you was to love you.
You made everyone better and everything brighter.
Your friendship is one of the greatest honors I'll ever receive.

This world just isn't the same without your light. May your selfless leadership, infectious laughter, and Beyoncé dance moves live on forever.

I love you beyond all of the clouds and stars in the sky.

2019

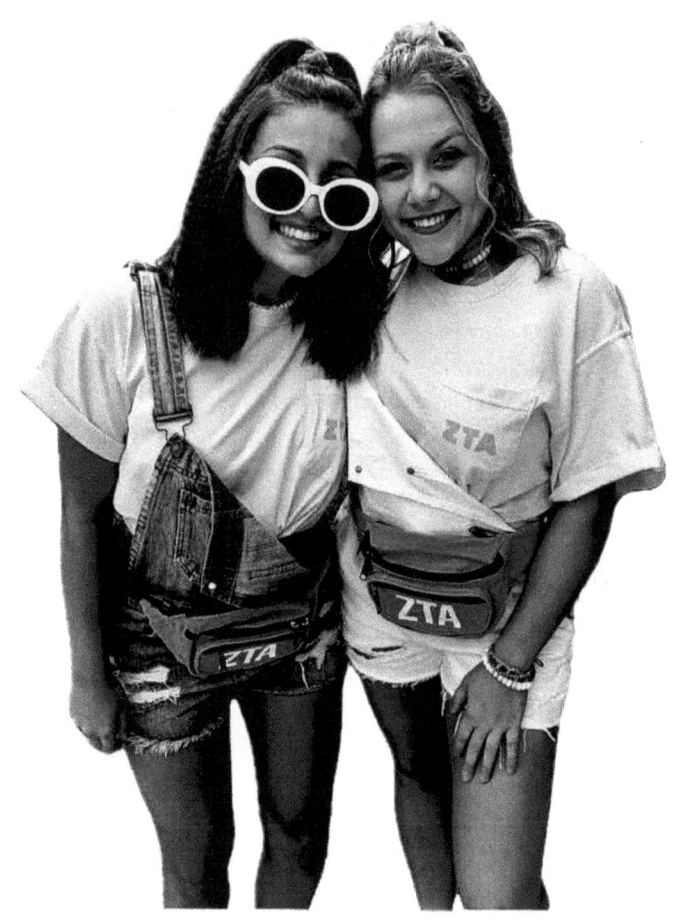

"Live your best life"
—Dom, the girl who continues to change the world

UNKNOWN WARRIOR

I am tired.

Tired of comparing others and criticizing myself.
Tired of trying to meet unrealistic standards and setting myself up for failure.
Tired of emotionally and physically putting my body through hell.

I am exhausted but I will carry on.

2019

When you reach a red light, you stop.
When your gas gauge is empty, you fill it.
My car even alerts me when I'm swerving.

We yield to signs and honk to stop accidents.

So why do we ignore these same signals in our own lives when it comes to our bodies and minds?

Someone please pull me over so I'm forced to stop, even if only for a minute.

Trigger Warning: Bulimia

I didn't realize I was developing a restrictive mentality. I didn't realize my constant limitations began the cycle that would fuel my binges. I didn't realize how easy it was for a night of eating to turn into a night of purging.

One of my first "episodes" was over half a sandwich. Half a sandwich that maybe totaled less than a quarter of the calories I should consume in a day. Half a sandwich that, when you break it down, are carbs, dairy, some fat, and a vegetable (or fruit, depending on which team you think tomatoes are on).

I felt regret as soon as I picked it up. I felt the sandwich hit my stomach before I even swallowed it. I felt guilty for secretly enjoying the taste of real food. I felt ashamed and relieved knowing I could "get rid" of the calories once I was finished.

Looking back with more clarity, I realize now that I was more in control than I felt at the time.

I wish I had the strength to tell myself: *You can fight this. You do not have to surrender to regret, guilt, and shame. Bulimia is a slippery slope. It's an eating and mental disorder. It's a coping mechanism and it's an addiction. But it does not define you.*

2019

You can overcome this. You can break the cycle. You can get to the light at the end of the tunnel. Your life is worth so much more than silent, tearful nights on your bathroom floor. Your body and mental health are worth too much to destroy. YOU are worth too much to destroy. You are resilient and I believe in you.

*I have been going back and forth trying to find the words to say this. This page holds a heavy place in my heart because it talks about one of my hardest journeys . . . one that I am still on. I am able to share and accept my experience because of the help I have received through years of therapy. If you struggle with anything mentioned above, I encourage you to reach out for help from a trusted professional.

Abandoned.

*A feeling I know all too well and a word that sends chills
down my spine.*

2019

Let's ask ourselves the hard question:

Why are we so afraid of gaining weight?

When my disordered eating was at its worst, I had a million reasons to justify why extra pounds were the worst thing that could possibly happen to me:

- My favorite pair of jeans would fit me differently.
- People would think I was ugly.
- I'd never stop gaining weight.
- I'd lose my image of being a "fit girl."
- I'd be "unhealthy," unhappy, and unlovable.

And then it all hit me.

I wasn't afraid of physically buying different jeans, but afraid someone would notice I outgrew my old ones.

I wasn't afraid of losing my image, but afraid of the new words someone would use to describe me and my bigger body.

I wasn't even afraid of being "unhealthy" at all. I knew what I was doing was wrong. I knew I wasn't physically or emotionally okay. But being "skinny" was more important to me than, well, anything else.

In fact, what I was absolutely terrified of was recovery. I didn't know what life was like beyond an eating disorder and couldn't picture a life without one.

I convinced myself that if I were smaller, I'd be happy. I'd be so beautiful. I'd be lovable. Contrary to everything we are told, your happiness, beauty, and worth do not come from your reflection in the mirror.

Be honest with yourself, what are you truly so afraid of?

My cup is empty and I keep trying to pour every nonexistent drop out of it as if it won't notice there's nothing left.

You can't pour from an empty cup.

2019

June 5, 2019: my eating disorder recovery anniversary.
A day I will always feel proud, exhausted, hopeful, and every emotion in-between.

Write the person who hurt you the most in this world a letter, even if it is yourself.

A letter to release your feelings.
A letter to accept all that happened.
A letter to forgive them or one to say you don't know if you ever will.

Let your feelings and words flow.

Happy writing, my love. I'll see you on the other side.

Journal Prompt 2.0

2019

You were wrong about me.
You crossed a line time and time again.

I still wince when someone turns the corner carrying the same energy you did.
I still find pieces of you in new people I meet.
I still remember moments from years ago like they were yesterday.

I forgive you, but your words are burned on my heart.

I don't know if I will ever forget them.
I don't know if I've completely worked through this.
I don't know if I ever will.
But I do know I am done spending my life trying to prove to you I was enough all along.

Part of my letter.

I wish you fought for me.

But I can't thank you enough for not doing so. Because it gave me a chance to fight for myself.

To all the foes in my battle that made me an unknown warrior.

2020
the year of never-ending uncertainties

Nutrition Intake Form
Completed on January 28, 2020, at 10:29 p.m.

Tell me about the primary purpose of our meeting. What exactly led you to make this appointment?
I reached my breaking point the day before I was set to return to college after winter break. I was afraid to come back to this environment and be surrounded by a culture heavily focused on what you look like. I stepped on the scale and gained two pounds in one week after following Weight Watchers and going to the gym. I was in hysterics, so I took the initiative/leap of faith to ask for help.

Have you seen a dietitian before?
It was a very negative experience. Her restrictive plan and unsympathetic mindset led me to binge and purge. My mind is now flooded with different plans, and I need to bring my body back to its equilibrium. I am frustrated and I put my body through hell. I am trying to make progress, but it is hard because my body is reacting to all the sudden and aggressive changes I have made. I genuinely don't know how to get better but am willing to try and learn.

What are your top goals for our work together?
My goal is to feel better. I have been fighting this battle for as long as I can remember and I want to feel like I have some control back in my life. I am hoping to build a better relationship with food. I have been sucked into so many unrealistic diet trends and I want to learn the truth about a healthy lifestyle.

If you had a magic wand and could change something in your life, what would it be? What does that ideal picture look like?
If I could change one thing, I would allow myself to take a deep breath. I tend to go from 0-100 and I feel like I am walking on eggshells with my anxiety and perfectionist tendencies. I would use my magic wand to feel confident in every aspect of my life. I would feel better and happy.

Where would you like to see yourself one year from now? Five years from now?
One year from now I am hoping I have a better control over my emotions, anxiety, and life. I feel like I am currently in a situation I can't do much about. In five years, I can't even imagine where I'll be. I just pray that I am happy and no longer revolve my life around my acne, weight, or physical appearance.

Is there anything else you feel is important to mention?
This has taken over my life. I am exhausted and scared to try again because if this doesn't work, I would be broken. I struggle with anxiety, acne, body image issues, and eating disorder tendencies. These all go hand in hand, so when it rains it pours. I know what it's like to feel better, and it was the best thing that has ever happened to me and I would do anything to feel that way again.

I wish the girl filling out this form could see me now, exactly 3 years and 2 weeks from the moment she submitted this . . . Healthy, in Rome, eating with lifelong friends who were only strangers a few weeks ago (keep reading for the Italy stories hehe). I wish she knew that the broken feeling she felt so deeply in that moment wouldn't last forever. I wish I could tell her that she was strong enough to make it through every single battle she would face.

After submitting that form, I began working with a certified eating disorder dietician: Erica. During our first session, she told me:

"I cannot say if you will gain, lose, or maintain your current weight. But what I can tell you is that whatever happens is supposed to. If you gain, you are getting closer to a healthy weight that you will be able to maintain."

That is the first time I heard that your body is intended to be a certain size.

What a concept?!

Your "ideal weight" is the one where you feel strong and energetic, where you feel your best regardless of appearance. It's a weight you can maintain effortlessly, without adhering to a strict diet or rigorous workout routine.

If you listen to your body about how to nourish and move it, everything will fall into place. Your body will guide you home.

Erica also introduced me to the concept of "food exposures." This practice involves a profound shift in mindset—it's about confronting and enjoying the foods you've long avoided, but with a new perspective. It's not a matter of cheating or burning off calories; it's about embracing food for what it truly is.

Building a healthy relationship with food starts by challenging our subconscious beliefs. We need to stop categorizing food as "good" or "bad" and end the cycle of tying our self-worth to what we eat. Recently, I've been pushing my boundaries with food exposures. I order acai bowls, pastas, sandwiches, and casual cocktails—not as indulgences to be punished, but as balanced meals to be enjoyed.

Food fuels our bodies and nourishes our spirits. It creates moments of connection, like sharing a charcuterie board and pear arugula salad with a best friend. The emotional and social benefits of eating are often overlooked, but they're just as crucial as the nutritional aspects.

Food exposures offer freedom from guilt, allowing us to experience joy instead of shame. I promise you the foods you are running away from are not as scary as you make them out to be.

This is no easy task. You are rewiring your brain from years of consistent thoughts. It is normal to feel intimidated. It's challenging and requires hard work. But guess what? It's worth it. And the more you do it, the easier it gets.

You've got this. I know you do.

2020

For me, food freedom is impulsive Italian dinners in an XL sweatshirt with no makeup on.

Food freedom is enjoying the bread before your meal no matter what you ate earlier in the day (and yes, always dunk it in the olive oil and balsamic).

Food freedom is ordering the rigatoni anyway.

Food freedom is eating tiramisu even when you convince yourself it's "not necessary."

I went to dinner with my roommate, Gwen, and ordered REAL fettucine with REAL Alfredo sauce.

She could sense my hesitation before I ordered and reminded me that the Earth doesn't care enough to base its rotation off of what I choose to eat for dinner. She reminded me how insignificant our meals are in the grand scheme of things.

Why do we continue to place the weight of the world on them?

Why do we let them hold so much value?

At the end of the day, a restrictive mentality will truly do more damage to our bodies than a bowl of noodles ever will.

Eat foods that scare you. Let yourself enjoy the moment—and while you're at it, listen to "Pasta" by New Rules.

My first food exposure.

Although the light at the end of the tunnel may seem dim right now, it is important to remember it will always be there.

Not knowing what the next few months have in store has me thinking. Before I left for spring break, I didn't hug my friends as tight as I should have because I knew I would see them in a week. I didn't soak in driving around Narragansett because I couldn't wait to get away and I knew I'd be back. All the constants I had in my life changed in an instant. The little things I took for granted and the big things I thought would never change are all in limbo. It puts everything into perspective. It reminded me that sometimes we do things for the last time and never know it.

Through all the uncertainty, I can't help but feel grateful—so unbelievably grateful for all the times I *did* have and for how much more I will appreciate them in the future.

It is rare we get a chance to reconnect and recharge.
It's time to stop—to take a step back and finally breathe.
It's time to find beauty in the stillness.
It's time to hold onto every ounce of love you can.
It's time to take care of yourself, those around you, and know better days are coming.

The Global Reset: March 13, 2020

2020

For me, one of the hardest parts of recovery has been old photos—they are my triggers.

I look back on some pictures and it makes me sad. Sad because I can see right through my smile. Sad because I can still hear all the hurtful things I was telling myself. Sad because I can even remember the number on the scale from that morning before the photo was taken, and I know it was much lower than it is now.

I find myself wishing I could go back to certain moments and say:

Relax your shoulders.
Stop sucking in.
Your friends love you!
Enjoy where you are—one day you will give anything to go back.

I vow . . .
To never again miss out on a second of this precious life because of my weight.
To never again think that I'd be happier if I was living in a different body.
To never again look at a photo and say, "Look at how beautiful I was."

Because I still am and always will be.

A picture is a moment in time,
and if it's posted on Instagram . . . it's probably edited.

My acne scars make me, me; I wouldn't change them for the world.

Adult acne is not only normal, but beautiful.

2020

A series of letters I sent to an inpatient eating disorder recovery facility

To you,

The average person has 60,000-80,000 thoughts a day. Make sure a good chunk of them today are reminding yourself that you are worth it. I hope 2021 is the start of something great. I hope it is when you learn that your body is your best friend. I hope it is when you finally find a home within yourself. I am thinking of you!

Sending so much love, as a stranger.

Xo
Sar

UNKNOWN WARRIOR

To you,

If you are worried that it will always be this way, here is your reminder that it will get better one day soon. You are beautiful, you always have been. But you are meant and made for so much more than that. You are strong enough to be your own hero, and that is something to be proud of. So, hang in there, because there is so much waiting for you on the other side of this. I am cheering you on!

Warm thoughts from someone you don't know.

Xo
Sar

2020

To you,

Whenever you are at your lowest, remember the last time you were there and all you've accomplished since then. Remember that you aren't broken; you are breaking *through*. Remember that sometimes all you can do is take a deep breath and keep going. Remember that you are loved beyond words. You are doing one of the greatest things you will ever do for yourself. I am so proud of you.

Sending kind thoughts your way, even though we've never met.

Xo
Sar

UNKNOWN WARRIOR

To you,

Today, think of all that you are instead of all that you are not. Don't only think about, but *believe* how much more beautiful the world is with you in it. There is a past you out there who is overflowing with so much pride looking at how far you've come. In case you can't feel it for yourself at this moment, know that I believe in you. Catch my hug!

From one stranger to another, sending love and strength.

Xo
Sar

2020

To you,

I promise you, it gets better. And sometimes you just have to hang onto that cliché quote with everything you have in you. A bad day does not take away from how far you've come. I know you will beat this. You are stronger than that little voice in your head telling you, you can't. And even if you can't see that right now, know that I do and am rooting for you.

Sending so much love from someone who cares but doesn't know you.

Xo
Sar

When I was eight years old, I first learned about eating disorders. Although I didn't fully understand them, I remember feeling a deep sense of helplessness.

I saw my little cousin, Mali, for the first time in a long time. She ran up to me and exclaimed, "Sar!! I'm eight now!!"

A lump formed in my throat, and tears welled up in my eyes. I hugged her tightly, and when she noticed my tears, I told her she is enough just as she is, and that will never change. She looked at me curiously, gave me another hug, and then we spent the evening laughing together.

The thought of Mali ever feeling inadequate, hating her body or her reflection, avoiding certain foods or time with friends, and criticizing herself breaks my heart. It pains me even more knowing that someone close to me struggled with these challenges at such a young age.

Today, I encourage you to connect with your inner child. Give them the hug they deserve and, when you find it hard to love yourself, imagine offering those same words and love to your little self, with their whole life ahead of them. It will make the journey a little easier.

2020

It's time for a book break!

Get comfortable in your chair.
Close your eyes.
Take five deep breaths.
List three things you are thankful for.
Think of one small thing you will do for yourself today and plan to make it happen.
Look away from the pages and up at the world around you.
One more breath.

Okay, continue.
Happy reading!

They say you only get a handful of special moments in your life. You know, the ones where you realize how badly you are going to miss it while you're living it? The ones where you just know while it's happening that you're going to remember it for the rest of your life?

But here's the thing. I think those moments are much more frequent than we make them out to be. I think we tend to think of everything that could happen next or everything that could go wrong so we wind up missing the moment all together. I think if we just make space for them, if we let them happen, if we get out of our own way and let ourselves enjoy it ... we'll see the next miracle is right around the corner.

So, stop telling yourself no. Stop coming up with reasons why you can't. Stop saying you're too busy without even looking at your schedule. Stop blaming your body. Sure, adulting is hard, but so is watching life pass you by.

Jump in the water with your clothes on. Who cares if you're a little cold on the walk home? You'll dry.

Leave your job if you hate it as much as you say you do—and while you're at it, move down to that city. What's the worst that happens? You can always find your way back home.

Go get the tattoo. I think if there's meaning behind it, you'll never fully regret it.

Pop the bottle of champagne, order the pancakes, and don't you dare waste time looking in your mirror with unkind eyes.

And if you've made it this far reading this, go do it.

You know? The thing that popped into your head . . . that thing you're thinking of right now? The sign you've been waiting for . . . this is it, my dear!

How about we stop saying it is partly cloudy and say it is mostly sunny?

I've been catching myself wishing I had a different body.

One that was smaller.
Fitter.
Just "better."

And then I thought, *Better for who?* And more importantly, *Why?*

Why would I want to drown myself in thoughts around food and exercise to live in a body I'm clearly not meant to have?

Why should I seek validation from others based on an idealized "transformation"?

Why can't I be happy with the body I have right now, at this very moment?
Why can't I?
Why can't you?

2020

Life is short. Too damn short.

The truth we know but often forget.

They say you learn something new every day. At Friendsgiving, I learned a lot.

I learned that food freedom is a beautiful thing. That drinking wine for no reason and eating food without working for it feels really good.

I learned I'll never be able to make my mom's mac and cheese as good as she does (the secret is throwing crumbled Cheez-Its on top before it goes in the oven).

I learned eating disorder recovery is powered by baby steps and that you can break any disordered habit if you set your mind to it.

I learned you're way stronger than you give yourself credit for.

I learned you don't need to restrict, binge, or purge.

I learned worrying about what you look like is an utter waste of time.

I learned that you should keep going, because you may be almost there and not even know it.

I learned when you're in a room full of people who love you, what you ate all day or what you're wearing doesn't matter at all.

I learned I love making/eating charcuterie boards, and dinner parties are a great way to spend your 20s.

I learned people are more inspired by the real you: the one who struggles and has flaws. That the light you see in everyone else is shining in you as well. That you have the ability to change a stranger's life, and that is not something to take lightly.

I learned just how thankful I am for this time in my life.

2020

More than anything, I learned one day all the hardships you went through will be worth it. That there is so much love in the world. And, sometimes, a darker tunnel makes it even easier to see the light at the end of it.

I learned that with all of the uncertainty this year has brought, it is important to hold on to and appreciate your constants.

I think you should keep learning, just to see what happens.

Your body is an archive of experiences.
It is meant to take you to amazing places.
It is meant for creativity, relaxation, and enjoyment.

Your body is designed to savor a wide variety of foods.
It is made to fix your broken bones and heal your wounds.
It is made to dance with your friends.

Your body's sole purpose is to keep you alive, that's all it has to live for.
It was made to wrinkle.
It is supposed to grow and shrink to support you through the different stages of your life.

Your body was put on this earth to do so much goodness, not look like someone in a magazine.

2020

Coffee isn't breakfast.
Lunch is a very important meal.
It's never too late at night to eat dinner.

And for the love of God, can we please get rid of the negative connotation around snacking?

Normalize eating six meals a day if that's what your body needs.

I am the only one who can pick myself up.

But sometimes I don't even have the energy to stand.

Being hungry isn't wrong.
Eating right after you have a meal isn't wrong.
Having lunch an hour before you're "supposed to" isn't wrong.

Who convinced us it was?

Have you ever heard someone say . . .

"If you aren't hungry for an apple then you definitely aren't hungry for a cookie."

I have, all the time actually. Come to think of it, I know a lot of people that ENCOURAGE this mentality.

But here's where that logic is flawed:

Maybe you aren't hungry for an apple because you already had a serving of fruit and haven't eaten enough carbs. Maybe you've been depriving your body of sweets for a few days. Maybe eating is a lot simpler than we make it out to be.

When you want to deny your hunger, ground yourself and ask:

When did I last eat?
Was it a meal or a snack?
Did I get all my food groups in?

Please do not destroy your mental health and diminish your self-worth over a few fats and carbohydrates.

Listen to your body and give it what it needs.

2020

I forgive you for the comments you made about my body when you were struggling with yours.

I forgive you for the things you said when you were uneducated on eating disorders.

I forgive you for looking at me differently knowing I was prescribed anxiety medication.

I have found peace within myself to truly forgive you, to wish nothing but the best for you and to thank you . . .

I am stronger because of you.

The truest form of closure comes from within.
A letter I wrote to forgive people in my past.

Every week I ask my therapist, Jenny, for "homework." and every week she laughs. Sometimes recovery just seems to be too much, so I break it down and focus on one thing to work on.

One week, my homework was to feel joy. To do whatever I wanted. Or, for that matter, not to do something. So, I'm assigning this to you.

Have the fries if you don't want a side salad.
Go for a walk if your body doesn't feel up for a workout.
Stay in for the night if you need to recharge your social battery.
Reach out to an old friend if you miss them.
Order an iced coffee with all your favorite flavors added to it.
Celebrate a random night out for no reason at all.
Wear the outfit you feel most confident in.
Go somewhere. Say something. See someone.

When was the last time you did something for you and only you?

It's probably been a while.

This week, do something because you actually want to. Not because it's what everyone else is doing or you think it's what you should be doing. Do it because it will bring you the overwhelming happiness you deserve.

You'll never get to do today again, so let's do it right. Happy (whatever day it is)!!!!!

2020

I wish I could go back to the last time I had brunch with my girls.

I would've ordered the lemon ricotta pancakes instead of the egg white veggie omelet.

I would've enjoyed the food I was eating, rather than worry about how many calories were in it.

I would've laughed. I would've listened. I would've let go. I would've let myself feel the love around the table.

I would've told myself to stop worrying, stop overthinking, and to start living.

From now on, I will take a breath, cherish those around me, and soak in everyday for all that it is.

I cannot wait to eat and ENJOY IT . . .
And I am so excited for breakfast potatoes with extra hot sauce.

Brunch is the most important meal of the day.

UNKNOWN WARRIOR

If all you've done today is make it through, you've done more than enough.

And I'm proud of you for it.

When you're cold, you feel like you'll never be warm again.

When you're tired, you feel like you'll never be energized again.

When you're sick, you feel like you'll never be healthy again.

When you're sad, you feel like you'll never be whole again.

When you are full, you feel like you'll never be comfortable again.
But you will.
Your body will digest everything you ate. You will not be in pain. And you will be at ease before you know it.

A reminder for when your intrusive thoughts are just too loud.

UNKNOWN WARRIOR

When it comes to choosing your partner and romantic relationships . . .

Nah, this isn't the book for this hahaha.

Hold your head high and your standards higher.
Set healthy boundaries and be kind.
Love whoever you want and love them proud.

That's all I got on that.

2020

Things we should stop doing:
Skipping meals.
Sucking in.
Purging.
Pushing our bodies past the point of pain.
Making ourselves more "desirable."
Trying so damn hard to make someone fall in love with what's on the outside.
Doing everything in our power to morph our bodies, change our personalities, and fit ourselves into these molds we were never supposed to be in in the first place. All of this so we will feel worthy enough for . . . a partner!?

I'm not sure about you, but I'd rather:
Smile big and laugh loud.
Dance like nobody's watching.
Move and fuel my body as needed.
See myself as more than a to-do list of things to fix.

I'd rather live as my unapologetic self. I'd rather attract someone I don't need to wear a "mask" for. I'd rather fill my life with people who don't need convincing that I'm good enough as I am.

You don't have to jump through hoops. You were worthy of love yesterday, you are worthy of love today, and you will be worthy of love tomorrow.

There is no need to change who you are to make room for someone else in your life. All of the love you need is already inside of you . . . a partner is just a bonus.

For the gals.

You are so much more than what you struggle with inside.

And I am so sorry society made you feel you had to hide.

For the guys.

It's a Friday night back at college. I hope you have fun. I hope you are safe. But more than anything, I hope you stop.

I hope you stop being told "pulling trig" (a.k.a. puke) and rallying will make you feel better. And I hope your friends stop offering to do it for you.

I hope you don't have to hear about how little someone ate all day or how they skipped a meal so they "wouldn't have to drink as much to get drunk."

I hope no one comments on your body or gives you unsolicited advice.

I hope you stop pinching your body, criticizing yourself, and staring at your reflection in the mirror until you find something you don't like. I hope you stop wishing for better clothes, better hair, better skin, and a better body.

The outfit your friend is wearing, the girl on Instagram, the guy at the bar, the dinner you ate . . . I hope you know none of it matters.

The people around you. The music you dance to. The way you feel about yourself. Your happiness, your memories, your health. You . . . THAT is what matters.

I hope you feel beautiful tonight. I hope you are kind to yourself.
I hope you believe you wouldn't have more fun if you took up less space.
I hope you feel genuine happiness tonight and every Friday after, because you deserve it.

For the college kids.
Man, I'm old.

There is a difference between exercising in ways you enjoy and pushing yourself beyond limits to "earn the right to eat."

There are different needs for every single body on this planet.

There is often necessary weight needed to gain in eating disorder recovery.

There is no way for you to tell someone's health status just by looking at them.

It's not about gaining weight.
It's not about losing weight.
It's not about going or not going to the gym.

It's about your mental and physical health.
It's about being comfortable in your own skin and learning there is so much more to life than what you look like.
It's about finding love within yourself instead of your reflection in a mirror.

I don't owe you an explanation for the way my recovered body looks or for the choices I make about how I eat and move.

For the people who just don't get it.

Interrupting your reading with some much-needed reminders:

You weren't born hating your body.

Food is meant to have calories because:
Calories. Are. Energy.

The happiest you've ever been won't be the happiest you'll ever be.

Restriction works . . . until it doesn't—and I promise you it won't work forever.

Social media is a highlight reel.

An eating disorder will do more harm to your body than a bowl of pasta ever will.
(Please read that sentence again.)

Weight loss won't fix a negative body image.

Your body is your home, not a to-do list of things to "fix."

It's not going to be easy, but it'll be worth it.

You are stronger than your struggles.

You always have and always will be enough.

Final reminder until I let you get back to reading: you'll never get this moment back again, so don't waste it away wishing you were anyone else but yourself.

Have you ever looked in the mirror and thought . . .

I wish I could just literally chop [insert part of your body you dislike] *off!*

My dear, why on earth would you want to get rid of something that makes you . . . you?

Journal Prompt 3.0

2021
the year I began to pick up the pieces

For years, I labeled myself as the "bigger friend."

I said it so much I not only let it skew my perception of myself, but I let it become a piece of my identity. As my eating disorder developed, I felt the need to compensate for being the "bigger friend" and make sure they saw me as "worthy" in other ways.

So, I tried to become . . .
The "food-and-workout-obsessed" friend.
The "loud Italian" friend.
The "therapist" friend.
The "fun (and occasionally drunk)" friend.
The "overachiever" friend.

Looking at it from 10,000 feet up, I'm able to see there was no need to label myself at all. I'm just me: their friend and that has always been more than enough.

Your friends love you because of who you are, not because of what you do or what you look like. They love you because of the way you make them feel. When you surround yourself with people who see you for who you are beyond the surface, it makes you feel like you can fly. It makes you feel undoubtedly worthy.

Next time you feel anxious about your size, remember it's okay to take up space. It's okay to be the bigger friend. It's more than okay to show up exactly as you are.

You are you and that is your superpower. Your friends love you just as you love them. Don't forget to remind them and yourself of it today!

> *Now I just want to be the friend that makes my people feel safe and loved.*

2021

You do not need to burn off what you eat.
You do not need to exercise to deserve food.
You do not need to justify your body to anyone. Ever.

I am so sorry you were made to feel that you did.

I am not underweight, but I am not okay.

I am struggling with an eating disorder and I am deserving of help,
no matter my size.

2021

Disgusting.
Everything they said about you was true.
You failed.

I have been constantly replaying these thoughts in my mind.
I haven't felt like myself in a long time.
I didn't realize the damage I had done or how unbelievably destroying my self-talk was.

Umm . . . *failed*? That's pretty freaking brutal, don't ya think? As harsh as it was, I convinced myself I was a failure and I reminded myself of it every single day.

I dug deep. I let my guard down, looked at myself with grace, and for the first time in a long time, I was able to see myself for who I was, not what I looked like.

I saw the girl who was hurting so deeply.
The girl who was doing her best to hang in there.
The abandoned girl, who was angry, frustrated, and sad that I turned my back on her.

I saw the girl who needed a hug, a deep breath, and a break.
The girl who KNOWS Dom would be so sad to see her like this.
The girl who has lived through the hell I put her through.
The girl who never fails to show up to fight the same relentless uphill battle.
The girl who deserves to strut around in a two-piece bathing suit, no matter her size.
The girl who is so much more than what she looks like and deserves so much more than what I have given her.
The girl who deserves to be loved: acne scars, cellulite, round stomach, and all.
The girl who should never let anyone talk down to her, including herself.

I looked in the mirror and saw the girl who is done being the victim of her own thoughts.

Oh, you think I've failed? This is what failure looks like to you? Well, keep watching, because my favorite thing to do is prove people wrong, even if it's myself.

STEP AWAY FROM THE MIRROR, DRINK A BIG GLASS OF WATER, AND EAT SOMETHING THAT MAKES YOU FEEL GOOD.

You don't need my permission, but I understand the desire for it.

You did it.
You stopped comparing yourself to others. You've heard it hundreds of times and it finally clicked.

But there's still a small piece of you that feels like you are inadequate.

Maybe it's not only others you compare yourself to.
Maybe it's a lot deeper than that.
Maybe we need to stop comparing ourselves to . . . ourselves.

It's so easy to look back and compare yourself to the "best self" you've ever been.
The time you had clearer skin.
The time you wore that dress.
The time everything unexpectedly fell into place.

It's no wonder why we always feel like we are falling short of what we "should be."

Instead of comparing ourselves to our old physical being, let's take a minute to look deeper. If you are going to think about your "old self," think about how you made it to the light at the end of the tunnel that you couldn't even see before. How you made it through the thing that you never thought you could. The you who never thought they would get to where you are now.

It's time to stop comparing and evaluating all together. Let's appreciate and love who you are today, because you will never be this you again. If you ask me, the you, the one you are right now, is pretty damn great.

Sometimes all you need is a little faith in the universe and in yourself that things will work out exactly as they are supposed to.

When it comes to your body:

- Trust that it has your best interest in mind.
- Listen to what it needs.
- And on the days where you can't love it, accept/appreciate it for all that it is.

How I think of it in four steps?

1. respect your body
2. accept your body
3. like your body
4. love your body

When you find yourself struggling to like your body, remember that acceptance is a solid foundation you can fall back on. This way, even if you stumble, you're not starting from scratch but rather building from a place of understanding and respect.

My stepladder of self-love.

"I know it was hard at times but you made it like everyone knew you would and I hope you made some memories along the way. You're probably nervous right now to go out into the real world, but you got this and I'm so proud of you. You didn't come this far to only come this far. Peace out URI, the real world is lucky to have you. Here comes the pain.

Love, Sar"

A letter I opened the morning I graduated college:
From Freshman Year Sar to Senior Year Sar

We have more conversations with ourselves than we do with any other person in this lifetime. So let's not only be kind with our words but be our biggest hype-man.

There is so much good coming your way and you deserve every ounce of it. Create space for it, allow yourself to experience it; let it all in. Above all else, enjoy it. There was a time not too long ago that you wished for everything you have now.

You are strong. You are radiant. You are effortless. You are worthy.

You're a fighter. You're growing. You're powerful. You're a dream.

You are someone's hero.
You make this world a brighter place.
You are one beautiful badass.

You are a superhero.

Instead of waiting for the light at the end of the tunnel, use your self-love superpowers to light that bitch up yourself. Everything you need is already inside of you; all you have to do is believe it.

I hate the way you tear yourself apart when you see another person walk by.
I hate the way you notice so many good things about them but can't seem to find any in yourself.
I hate that you don't see all the people admiring you because you are too busy admiring them.
I hate that you have no idea how incredible and wonderful you really are.

I hate this.
And I know Dom would've hated it too.

When you start gaining healthy weight, you may start to worry if you'll ever stop.

When you start allowing yourself to eat, you may start to panic that you've lost all control.

When you stop exercising, you may convince yourself you'll never start again.

The human body is an amazing thing. YOUR body is an amazing thing. All it wants to do is maintain a healthy homeostasis—and all we do is try and mess it up.

Your body will not let you down.
Listen to it and trust it.
Feed it and move it in ways that feel good.

It is then you will stop bingeing because you will have stopped restricting.
It is then your body will have energy so you will enjoy moving it.
It is then you will feel not only comfortable in, but grateful for the body you have.

You WILL get to that place. That place where you feel dynamic and strong. That place where you won't have to keep up with a strict diet or vigorous workout schedule to maintain your current weight. That place where you can have a glass of wine "just because" and eat a slice of cheesecake without "making up for it" the next day.

That place where you can start living and realize there is so much more to life than what you have been allowing yourself to see.

The real you.
The person you are when no one is looking.
The person who is unapologetically themselves.

That is my favorite version of you.

Not the person who saw a lower number on the scale.
Not someone who fits into a smaller pair of jeans.
Not the person who just got into a relationship or bought a new outfit.
Not someone who is having a good skin day.

We convince ourselves if we just lose some weight, meet our significant other, clear up our skin, or buy new clothes, *then* we will be happy. But when you had all those things, it brought you temporary satisfaction at best. So why would that change now?

All these surface-level things will never make you feel whole. They will never bring you the overwhelming joy you deserve.

If you haven't completed your homework assignment from earlier, intentionally choose joy for today.

2021

In case you forgot to tell yourself today, you are incredibly beautiful . . . but it is the least interesting thing about you.

Really.

I could go on for hours admiring every little thing about you—none of which having to do with your appearance:

Your welcoming eyes.
Your infectious energy.
Your heart and authenticity.
The way you light up when you talk about something you're passionate about.
The way you make others feel.
The way you love yourself.

You are beautiful.

Yes, you.

But you are also the reason someone will smile today. You are the reason this earth is still turning. You are unparalleled. You are a miracle. You are enough.

Do not let any scale, breakout, or "imperfection" convince you otherwise.

REGARDLESS OF WHAT OR HOW MUCH YOU ATE LAST NIGHT, YOU ABSOLUTELY DESERVE TO EAT TODAY. FUEL YOUR BODY AND OWN THE DAY.

What I heard:
"I know it's hot out, but don't give up on your run. You gotta earn that lasagna later!"
"I'll just take a water pill so I look skinny after drinking this weekend."
"Wow, you really went from one extreme to the other with working out!"

What I wanted to say:
"I don't need to earn anything."
"At best, water pills are ineffective, and you should never put something into your body for the sole purpose of 'looking skinny.'"
"I listen to my body and move it in other ways because how I was exercising before wasn't healthy."

But what I said was nothing.
All these comments were made with good intention by people who love me. So instead of fighting it, I internalized it and let their words linger.

I want you to stop blaming yourself for getting to where you are right now. I want you to know that the negative body image, food guilt, and intrusive thoughts aren't your fault. Once I became aware of my surroundings, I realized that triggers were everywhere I looked. They appeared in various forms: ads on my phone, conversations with my family, and behaviors of my friends. It felt overwhelming and inescapable.

You didn't ask for this, and you certainly don't deserve to feel this way. Recovery begins with awareness—how you talk to yourself, how you interpret the conversations and media around you, and how you engage with your circle. Everything matters, and you are worthy of a healthier, more compassionate perspective.

One day, I went about my morning routine, just like I always do, but this time I set a timer.

After snoozing my alarm and scrolling through social media, I got out of bed and do what I do every single morning:

I checked my body.

When I was finally done staring at myself, my timer said 14:23.
For fourteen minutes and twenty-three seconds I analyzed, compared, and criticized every inch of my body.

Sometimes I'm disgusted at first sight. Other mornings I keep staring until I find something I don't like. The other day, I literally put on a bathing suit "just to see" what it would look like. On the rare occasion I "approve" of my body, I take pictures only to look back at them later on and not be satisfied with how I looked.

Wanna know the ways I could've spent those fourteen minutes and twenty-three seconds?

I could've gotten an iced coffee on my way to work.
I could've done a face mask.
I could've listened to "Unwritten" by Natasha Bedingfield three and a half times.
I could've caught up with one of my friends from home.
Literally sleeping for the extra fifteen minutes would've been more productive.

You see, fifteen minutes every day may not seem like much. But, let's be honest, the morning isn't the only time we body-check.

To consider the bigger picture of this means that, without fail, I spend at least an hour and forty minutes a week in front of my mirror, wishing I had any body other than my own. In that same hour and forty minutes I could've:

Gone to lunch downtown.
Gone for a drive and sat by my favorite place.
Read the rest of the book I started but never found time to finish.
Watched four episodes of *New Girl* and had a glass of Pinot Grigio with my roommates.

So let's break the cycle and stop body-checking. Let's start our mornings on a better note and create space for all these other things that bring us joy. And if we must look in the mirror, let it be a chance to admire the resilient, loved, and beautiful person staring back at us.

During my last month in Rhode Island, I made a promise to myself that I wouldn't say no (within reason, of course).

I wouldn't say no to brunch with my roommates because I didn't want a "real breakfast."

I wouldn't say no to an adventure because I didn't feel comfortable in my clothes.

I wouldn't say no to going out for an espresso martini because the calories in alcohol weren't "worth it."

This promise allowed me to say yes to so many things I would've immediately shut down before. I ate, I drank, I smiled, I laughed, and above all else, I lived. For the first time in a long time, I felt free.

I didn't spend my mornings looking in the mirror, analyzing every crevice.
I didn't spend my days at the gym.
I didn't spend my free time obsessing over food and the calories it contained.

A whole month of allowing myself to be free of the thoughts and behaviors that have consumed me for years. I thought my world would stop turning, but at the end of it all, my body was healthy, and my spirits were higher than they had ever been. Sure, sometimes my stomach felt fuller than normal, but so did my heart, and that is a feeling I could get used to.

Today, this week, this month, this year . . . Please give yourself permission to be free, even if only for an instance. Say yes, even if only for a moment.

And never say no to the joy you deserve.

The happiest month of my life.

2021

In most of my Instagram posts, you see a girl reminding others to give themselves a proud and happy hug. What you don't see is the aftermath.

Sometimes, once the camera goes away, my smile goes with it. I might sit on the floor, eyes closed, allowing myself to fully feel my emotions.

Sometimes, I stay there until I've let out every tear and released all my pent-up emotion. I hug my body, rolls and all. I take a really deep breath, a good look in the mirror, and think to myself...

You see that girl staring back at you?
She may be struggling right now, but she is one hell of a fighter.
She's not broken, even when she's hurting. In fact, she's about to have a breakthrough.

Moments like this get me thinking, *I'm not the only one who had a tough week.*
So the next time you find yourself staring teary-eyed at your reflection...

Be proud of the person looking back at you.
Admire them for all they are.
Accept them for all they're not.
Thank them for all they've done.
Have faith that there is so much left for them to do.
Know they truly are beautiful and are going to change the world someday.

Remind them that everything they need is already inside of them, and that it's okay if they don't always feel like it.
Remind them they've placed too much value on their body for far too long.
Remind them their body will never be the best or worst thing about them.
Even if you don't believe it in the moment, tell them you love them: they deserve unconditional self-love more than anything.
And, most importantly, don't forget to give them a hug—they need it.

2021

It is time to reclaim your power.

It's time to give it everything you got.

It's time to show your inner voice who is in charge and don't you dare back down.

You showed up to fight.

You are strong.

You will beat this.

Your eating disorder may have won the battle, but it will not win the war.

Take back your power and reclaim your place in this world.

Let's f*cking do this.

I saved myself.

2021

I once got a text from my high school field hockey coach whom I hadn't spoken to in years.

She said:

"Hi! I'm currently cracking up over here. Wasn't it you who came to a game crying because George O'Malley died? I see he is returning to *Greys* and I immediately thought of you—how are you?"

I remember that game, but I haven't given it much thought since then. Once the memory was brought up, it felt like it happened yesterday. I wonder how many other moments I've let slip away.

If your anxiety is a little too loud and your eating disorder is getting the best of you, let this be your reminder that you matter.

That someone who you may not even think of cares about you. That they want the best for you. That other people smile because of you the same way you smile because of them. That you have made an impact in ways you could never imagine.

I've said it before and I'll say it again: your struggles matter, your story matters . . . you matter.

There is so much love in the world—and more than anything, there is so much love in YOUR world, even if you can't always feel it . . .

. . . never lose sight of that.

We are trained to praise weight loss, no matter what it takes to get there, and to look down on weight gain, no matter the reason behind it.

What a flawed way to look at things?
What a boring world it would be if we all looked, ate, and worked out the same?

Your gym stats do not define you. To be clear, someone else's gym stats definitely do not impact you in any way. Next time you find yourself comparing your workout to someone else's Apple Watch, remember that health looks different on everyone, a smaller size will never make you truly happy, and your being means so much more than your body does.

My recent gym wins are very different from what they used to be. For the first time, I'm not interested in calories burned or my personal records. Instead, I'm showing up by myself, for myself, and THAT is a victory worth celebrating.

Moving slowly is better than not moving at all.

I was at a bar with my best friend—one who weighs much less that I do—when a grown man came up to me, unsolicited, and said, "Hey, don't worry. Maybe one day you will be as skinny as she is."

I stood there speechless.

To you, Mr. Sir,

> Your words hurt so deeply because they run through my mind every time I am with her. Hopelessly waiting for the day I wake up and look like her.
>
> Maybe one day I'll get to live in a world without any body expectations. Maybe one day you'll mind your damn business.
>
> Maybe, just maybe, I'm going to continue to live my big and bold life in my worthy and beautiful, recovered body.
>
> Maybe you're right, one day I might be skinnier . . . but you'll always be an uneducated piece of shit! Thank you very much!

Get your hand and opinion off of me.

TIME FOR A DANCE BREAK!

BLAST YOUR FAVORITE SONG
TAKE A BIG SIP OF WATER
AND DANCE YOUR BIG HEART OUT

I'LL SEE YOUR CUTE SELF WHEN YOU'RE DONE

I broke the "food rules" that were given to me by God knows who.
I felt so much guilt I couldn't take it.
I was willing to do anything and everything to make myself "feel better."

I sat on my floor with two roads ahead of me. The first one was tempting and dare I say comforting, even though I knew it was deceiving me. I could see the whole way down it and knew exactly where it'd lead me. It was the road I thought I wanted to go down—the one I've been down many times before but knew I shouldn't because I was worth more than that.

The other one, now that was the scary one. I couldn't see beyond the first step. I didn't know what would happen along the way, but I knew in my gut this was the road that would lead me home.

I thought giving in to my eating disorder habits would ease my anxiety. And they would ... for five minutes ... maybe fifteen if I was lucky. But what I didn't realize was eating disorder behaviors would do more harm to my body than a meal ever would.

Every single day you get to choose where you take your first step—and that is your superpower. When you are sitting there (at the table, on your floor, or in front of your mirror), I want you to find your reason to take the second road. I want you to find your reason to trust your gut and take your leap of faith. I want you to find your reason to choose recovery.

I hope you are able to do it for yourself. But if you can't ...

- Do it for your family whose love for you goes deeper than appearances.
- Do it for your best friend who would do anything to take an ounce of your pain away.

- Do it for the person who held the door for you while leaving that place just to put some good out into the world.
- Do it for the days ahead that will be brighter than you could ever imagine.
- Do it for the stranger who is rooting for you unconditionally.
- Do it for the future you who is so proud you took the first step on the second road, despite your fears and hesitations.

The only way out is through. One meal at a time. One body at a time. One day at a time.

And if you're looking for a stranger to cheer you on, she's right here and she wrote this book for you.

Breakfast
- Peanut butter and jelly sandwich with a banana
- Yogurt with fruit and granola
- Oatmeal loaded up with your favorite toppings (chocolate, flax seeds, peanut butter—literally anything)
- A smoothie with everything you can find thrown in it
- Eggs! Eggs! Eggs!
- Avocado toast with a sprinkle of chili flakes . . . don't you dare think of using "45 calorie" bread
- Breakfast burrito with eggs, cheese, and salsa
- Chia seed pudding topped with fresh berries
- Bagel with cream cheese and smoked salmon
- French toast with maple syrup and a side of fresh fruit

Lunch
- A frozen veggie burger with pre-made guacamole
- Kraft mac & cheese with chicken sausage
- A turkey sandwich
- Your favorite Trader Joe's find
- Grilled cheese sandwich with tomato soup
- Pasta salad with vegetables, your comfort protein, and a tangy vinaigrette
- Loaded nachos with cheese, beans, and salsa
- Chicken or veggie quesadillas with a side of sour cream and pico

Dinner
- Baked ziti
- Stuffed bell peppers with rice and ground beef or turkey
- Homemade chili with beans and cornbread
- Roasted chicken with vegetables and potatoes
- Teriyaki chicken or tofu with broccoli and rice
- Beef or veggie stir-fry with noodles
- Frozen meals (Amy's is a personal favorite)

- Breakfast for dinner—you can never go wrong with chocolate chip pancakes
- Your favorite take-out restaurant

And for dessert . . . eat what feels good to you!

A list of meal ideas for when eating is hard.

"You are a strong, determined girl who has made tremendous progress. You are going to be so successful, but do not determine your worth off of your success. I care about you so much, so when I say 'Please let me know how you're doing,' I mean it."

The final session with my college therapist, Karen.

I go to the gym and I push myself to my limits. I also take days for myself where the most I do is get myself an unsweetened iced tea.
I genuinely enjoy salads and cooking. I also love a good M&M McFlurry and ordering Chinese food.
I get my nails and eyelashes done. I also rock a real messy bun, have breakouts, and walk around braless with no makeup on.

I think you should fuel and move your body but not forget to rest it.
I think you should eat your vegetables but trade them in for a buffalo chicken sandwich if your body is craving it.
I don't think it's all or nothing. I don't think you need to choose to label yourself as one or the other.

I think you should stop underestimating yourself. I think you're more than that. I think you truly can have and be it all.

I believe in taking care of yourself physically, mentally, and emotionally, however you need to. I believe in health and beauty, but I also believe those two words mean something different to everyone.

I believe there are a lot more layers to you than you recognize. I believe you are stronger than this and you WILL find a balance.
I believe recovery is worth it and there is a beautiful life beyond your eating disorder.

Above all else, I believe today is a good day to have a great day.

Throughout this past year, I have revisited all my highs and lows. I thought about all of the bodies I've lived in, challenges I've faced and battles I've won.

I thought about why I started recovering in the first place and how I almost didn't because I couldn't shake the fear of someone thinking I "let myself go."

I am now learning that "letting myself go" meant letting go of emotions and worry. Letting go of grudges and perfectionism. I let go and trusted that things would get better. And before I knew it, they did.

What are you afraid to let go of right now, and why can't you bring yourself to release it?

Journal Prompt 4.0

2021

I've said it before and I'll say it again: social media is a highlight reel, and New Year's may just be the most aggressive reel of them all.

My REAL year in review. 2021 . . . gosh I don't even know where to begin . . .
I got two more tattoos.
I started my senior year of college.
Besides starting @sar.calla on Instagram, I didn't "accomplish" too much during quarantine.
I spent a lot of nights at Bon Vue (my Thursday night spot in RI), 21 Atlantic Ave, and the Ryan Center.
My weight fluctuated a lot.
I spent a lot of time feeling alone in a room full of people.
No, Grandma, I still don't have a boyfriend.
I moved to Atlantic City.
I finished my presidency for my sorority, Zeta Tau Alpha.
I brought Adam (if you know you know) to Fort Laudy and had the best spring break ever.
I worried way too much about what I looked like.
At the time, I didn't have a plan for after graduation.
I ate a lot of sushi and drank a lot of Jameson.
I hung up my jazz shoes after nineteen years of dancing.
I lost some people who I thought would be in my life forever, but I found a few who have made my world a better place.
I did a lot of things for the last time and had no idea.
Some days hurt like hell. Others felt like a dream.
I cried hard and laughed harder. I felt a lot of pain followed by so much love.

I think that's what New Year's is all about, or at least what it should be. All of the ups and all of the downs, because that's what life is really like.

I don't know about you, but I think it's admirable to be able to admit "things have been hard, but I'm still standing." I think that's something to be proud of. I think that's much more impressive than saying how perfect everything is all of the time.

So let's be kind to ourselves and everyone around us. No one—and I mean NO ONE—has it together all of the time. We are all trying to figure things out the best we can. We all fought battles this year. We all made it through.

Here's to doing that again and hoping this year is the best one yet.

2022
the year I took my leap of faith

What if when you stepped on a scale it measured something other than pounds?
What if it could show you how resilient you are?
Or how bright your smile is?
Or how much joy it brings your best friend to hear your laugh?
Or how much love and light you bring into the world?

All this scale (that we dread so much) has the capacity to do is measure your "body mass times its acceleration due to gravity"... yup... you read that right. That intellectual sentence is something we have revolved our entire lives around.

If this scale was able to measure things that actually mattered, you probably wouldn't be so nervous to step on it, would you? Because unlike your weight, your worth never fluctuates.

Maybe then I wouldn't mind being heavy.
Here is to overcoming our fear of gaining healthy weight, together.

2022

I looked down at my leg today and remembered the first time I noticed my cellulite.

I was around fifteen years old.
I got had just gotten home from dance practice, where I had spent hours looking at myself in the mirror, and I said to my mom, "I don't like the way I look in these tights. My legs look really weird. What are these bumps? No one else has them."

I will never forget running my fingers down my leg, feeling the indents and wondering how the heck they got there.
I was quick to not blame the lighting, outfit, or positioning of my leg. Instead, I turned all of my loathing inward. I blamed the dinner I ate and workout I missed. I just blamed myself. My "failure" of self.

Today, looking down at my leg, I am seeing something much different.
I see a strong muscle that has allowed me to do some pretty amazing things.
I see my little thigh dimple coming out to say hi.
I see my stretch marks . . . literally glowing in the sunlight.

More than anything, I see a leg. A part of my vehicle.
One of the least interesting things about me.

And damn, are they strong.
#celluLIT 2.0

Home is a funny place. It reminds you of where you've been and motivates the true you to get to where you want to go.

I have had my very best and very worst days in Rhode Island [even though I will always be a Jersey girl].

I find so much comfort in that. Maybe that's why the biggest piece of my heart will always be there.

A journal entry: August 18, 2021

2022

I drove here the day I graduated college.

I sat here the morning I found out my friend passed away.

I ate here whenever I got my favorite takeout.

I read here when I needed some peace.

I observed the stillness when the world was spinning around me.

I sang here when my favorite artist dropped their new album.

I go here when I'm not sure where else to turn. I use this place for whatever I need. This is one of the few places I can go and just let myself be. You can always find me here, at my safe haven. My place that has weathered every storm. My place that is still standing tall. My place that felt like home, when I couldn't find one in myself.

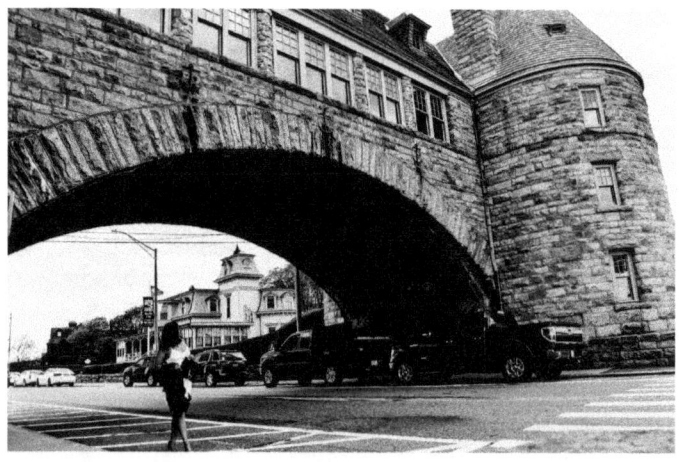

41.4305° N, 71.4556° W

Take a moment to reflect on what "home" means to you. For some, home might be a physical place. For others, home could be a person, a feeling, or a specific memory that brings comfort and belonging.

The Towers along the Narragansett Sea Wall is mine, where is yours?

Journal Prompt 5.0

2022

When faced with a tough decision, I often rely on my "Flip a Coin Theory." The idea is simple: when you flip a coin, deep down, you already know what you want it to land on. The coin flip isn't about leaving your fate to chance; it's about giving yourself a little push from the universe to validate what you already feel in your gut.

Here's how it works: flip the coin, but don't look at the result. Instead, pay attention to which outcome you're hoping for while the coin is in the air. That hope, that instinct, is your true answer.
So next time you're stuck, just flip a coin and trust your gut—you'll know what to do.

If it weren't for this, I may not have ended up in Rhode Island.

YOU DID NOT WAKE UP THIS MORNING TO HATE YOUR THIGHS AND BE ASHAMED OF YOUR STOMACH.

2022

I flew to Miami on a Tuesday just to spend nine hours in the sun with my roommate, Gwen.
I flew to Florida just to hug my friend Mirjana, who I hadn't seen in a year: I was there for one night.
I flew down south to celebrate Chris and Morgan's engagement for a day and a half.
I flew across the country to surprise Neen and spend thirty-one hours with her.
I flew to New Orleans with Al to celebrate seventeen hours at Mardi Gras.
I flew to Cleveland to go to a Machine Gun Kelly concert.
I flew to Bali with ten strangers and one of my idols, Juju.
I flew to Atlanta to see Chris Daughtry perform.
I flew from Boston to Philadelphia to get dinner with my family and leave the next morning.
I flew to New Mexico, Utah, and Illinois for weekend adventures because well . . . why not?

United 448
Delta 536
Delta 341
Delta 989
American 504
Delta 575
JetBlue 269
TK 82
TK 9368
JetBlue 900
Frontier 2287
American 2161
JetBlue 759

Book the dang flight.

A body that folds.
A body with rolls.
A body with a booty.

A body with curves, bumps, and wrinkles.

A body that has been through a lot.
A body that is recovering.
A body that is strong.
A body that is beautiful.

A body that has always been a bikini body.

A body that cannot wait to strut her stretch marks, cellulite, and acne scars around all summer.

My summer 2022 mood.

When you purge or use laxatives inappropriately, especially to try to lose weight, you're actually harming your body. Instead of achieving your goal, you're depleting essential electrolytes and stripping your body of vital water and minerals.

Another tool to add to your recovery toolbox: Rather than hyper-focusing on calories, simply realize they are just a calculation by how much energy it takes to break the food down. If calories were labeled as energy, would you then want the lowest number possible?

And a reminder that 100 calories to me is different from 100 calories to you.

I promise I will not make myself purge on this trip of a lifetime. I don't need it and my body deserves better than it. A year from now, what I ate won't matter but knowing I kept it all down will.

In my current recovery journey, I am living in a constant state of guilt and discomfort. I have recently surrendered myself to eating disorder behaviors and because of that, I am struggling to build trust within myself.

I've found breaking my goals into short-term "promises" helps me hold myself accountable. It gives me confidence to take the next step forward, even when I know there is a long road ahead. It provides a space for me to recognize and celebrate my little victories along the way.

Now, it's your turn.

I don't know about you, but my friends and I take our pinky promises very seriously, so make sure you pick something good; make sure you mean it.

Got it?

Okay, good.

Now hold it close to your heart.
Use it as your compass and let it ground you when things get tough. And, most importantly, believe you can keep it, because I know you can.

One day at a time and one promise at a time . . . we are capable of hard things. We can do this.

I'll hold up my end of the bargain if you do yours.

There's no going back on a pinky promise, so it looks like we are all going to do a little bit of healing today. I'm rooting for you, always—and I'll make you proud, I promise.

The power of a pinky promise.

2022

If you know me, you know I could easily live off of dumplings and unsweetened iced tea.

On our ridge walk adventure in Bali, I said to my new friend Amanda, "You know, I really wish someone was at the end of this hike just handing out dumplings."

We got to our destination (one of those restaurants where you take your shoes off when you walk in—which I was amped about), and I swear on all things good in this world . . . they brought out dumplings.

I wish words could fully capture how overwhelmed with happiness I felt—and still feel—because of those lil' dumplings. I should've played the lottery that day.

Man, do I miss Bali.
Stop #1 on my Eat, Pray, Love journey.

I used to restrict myself all day long . . .
"I can't eat that; I don't want to gain weight."
"I can't wear that; I am not thin enough for it."
"I can't go to that; I should stay in or go to the gym."

I convinced myself "I just couldn't."
I was "too busy," "too anxious," "too big."

Now . . .
I catch flights like it's my job and go on twenty-four-hour day trips every chance I can.
I wear clothes that make me feel good and enjoy the heck out of the food in front of me.

I am finally saying yes to the things I've always wanted to, and no jean size or number on a scale is going to stop me.

Here's your reminder to do the same and to enjoy every single day of your life.

2022

So,

If I'm not "big enough" to fit society's idea of a "desirable thick girl" . . .

And I'm not "small enough" to meet the standard of a "flawless thin girl" . . .

Then what the hell am I?

I'll tell you.
I'm someone who is going to label my damn self instead of letting others do it for me.

I'm Sar.
I'm me.
You can put me in any category you want, but I'm going to shatter any mold you try to confine me to.

I've learned it is more than okay to take up space. And I plan on taking up a whole lot of it. In my size, in my voice, and in my power.

A big bold and beautiful life awaits, my angel—
all you have to do is step into it.

Hear me out, my dear:
Your body has never been the problem.

Your body image is a deeply rooted, complex mindset which reflects how you "experience your embodiment." It has little to do with what your body actually looks like. This is why your body image changes on a day-to-day or hour-to-hour basis, even when your figure hasn't changed at all.

Your body is your home. It is your very best friend, even when it doesn't feel like it. It always has been and always will be enough . . . just as it is right now.

Your body is a masterpiece, deserving of admiration and love. Embrace it as the incredible work of art it truly is.

There is a missing piece inside of me: a sense of loss that doesn't have a name.
It is an emptiness I cannot shake.

My eating disorder was all-consuming. It didn't just influence my behaviors or thoughts; it controlled them.

It controlled me.

My eating disorder became the biggest part of me—the most sacred part of me. It was the only piece of my identity I understood. It was my safety blanket which allowed me to wear a mask. It was the version of myself I thought the world wanted to see.

My eating disorder was something I was proud of. I used to pride myself on being the girl who was obsessed with her food regimen and gym schedule. I used to be the girl who spent more time criticizing her reflection in the mirror than admiring the world around her. I used to be the girl who was driven by the idea of being as "perfect" as possible, no matter what it took to get there.

My eating disorder was more than I ever gave it credit for; it was all I ever knew.

I'd be lying if I said I didn't occasionally find myself missing my eating disorder and who I was when I was struggling most.
I'd be lying if I said I've never found myself missing my missing pieces that I know I shouldn't miss at all.

When I find myself struggling to accept/respect/like/love who I am without my eating disorder identity, I say: *Your missing pieces allow you to become who you really are. They allow you to start each day with a blank canvas and fill the gaps with the true you. They allow you to make space for the life you were meant to live . . . the life you deserve to live.*

I am coming to terms with the parts of me I've lost—and with that, I am coming into my own. I am coming into the light. I am becoming more than I ever could've dreamed of.

To my missing pieces . . .

. . . I am whole without you.

I started to fall off my path a little bit, and that is okay.
I was having trouble accepting my body, and that is okay.
I was struggling. I needed more help. I felt frustrated and lost, and that is okay.

When it comes to recovery, some days are a little harder than others, and that is okay.

You are trying to rewire your brain in a society that is consumed with diet culture. That is hard work. It is not only okay, but inevitable that you will have days where you want to throw in the towel.

Do you want to know what's not okay? Giving up.

Taking a moment to reflect, reset, and begin again does not mean you are starting back at square one. A difficult stretch of time does not take away from how far you've come. A lapse is not a relapse.

There is no roadmap when it comes to recovery. However you are feeling right now is okay. And it is more than okay if all you did today was survive.

Day by day, we're in this together.

When your world is spinning . . .
When your body is so tight you feel like you can't breathe . . .

Lay down, if you can. Close your eyes. And imagine yourself standing there.

Not your best-dressed self. Not you on a specific occasion. Just you, in your most comfortable state, standing there as you are. Get as clear of a picture as you possibly can.

Then, start to erase your body. From head to toe. Make sure you remove every single inch.

Your brain focuses so hard on creating the image and erasing every detail that it subconsciously calms your entire nervous system.

This tactic has gotten me through a lot. I hope it does for you too.

Thank you, Ms. Marge, for teaching us this during dance practice.

2022

It's a bump in the road. Not a dead end.

Relapses are sometimes a part of recovery.

You beautiful being,

I hear that little voice in your head, bargaining with you. Comforting you with your negative thoughts and magnifying our disordered habits. I know you care a lot about what they're saying and I know a small piece of you believes them.

If today is one of those days where your disordered thoughts feel a little too tempting, I want you to take a breath and read:

My smaller body brought me short-lived contentment. I still pinched, critiqued, compared, and ultimately hated my body. I was miserable. So why would a smaller pair of jeans make me happy now?

I missed out on so much life, and I don't plan on missing another second of it. I do not want to restrict myself anymore—I deserve so much more than that.

I am in control even when my disordered thoughts make me think otherwise. I show my true strength when I am kind to myself. I don't and never needed to binge, purge, or alter my body in any way.

My healthy body is a beautiful body.
My recovery is worth it.
I can do this.

Do not let that little voice in your head convince you otherwise.

2022

My body is growing. It is getting healthier and stronger every day.

But emotionally, I'm still withering away.

A tough day in recovery.

Remember the trend where you'd ask your friends, "What are three things I love?"

Every single person I asked responded with some variation of my eating disorder behaviors I masked as things that made me the happiest: reading food labels, TRX fitness classes, cauliflower rice, etc.

I fooled my closest friends; I even fooled myself at times. My eating disorder became such a normalized and prominent part of my identity that being thin, working out, and reading nutrition labels at the grocery store were things my friends thought I not only enjoyed, but loved doing.

Everyone wants to say goodbye to their eating disorder: they dream of it. But when it becomes a part of you—like a missing piece to a complicated puzzle called "YOU"—it's not as easy to walk away from.

Looking back on this trend a few years later, I came to find I'd much rather be the girl who loves drinking tequila and impulsive adventures than be the girl who is obsessed with her appearance and gym schedule. The person I have become is braver and more vibrant than any version of myself I've been before.

This step in my recovery is a place of unknown territory because a lot of people don't talk about this part . . . the messy middle. This shift in mindset happens suddenly and seemingly subconsciously. I have rejected food rules, turned my back on diet culture, and now I need to say goodbye to the (unhealthy) persona I worked so hard to create. I need to completely let go. I need to set myself free and I am the only one who can do it.

What do your people think you love the most?

2022

I used to wear smaller jeans and fake a smile. I liked having as many friends as possible. I would've never considered myself a leader. I didn't care for dumplings or feta cheese. I had longer, blonder hair. My camera roll was filled with "progress pictures" of my body. I was fighting a losing battle with myself. I was in denial and I was exhausted—but I never would have admitted it.

A few years ago, I decided I didn't want to be "that" girl anymore. I didn't want to be the girl who "does it all." It was only recently I learned how to break away from her. Rather than trying to be a superwoman for everyone else, I decided to be my own hero.

So Hi, I'm Sar!
But not the Sarah some of you may have gotten to know.

Why would you ever want to make yourself smaller? Reflect on the reasons for wanting to shrink your presence when you should be living life to the fullest and filling up the space you are in.

Journal Prompt 6.0

2022

2022, damn... where do I begin?
I wrote a book and released clothing merchandise.
I started volunteering with NEDA.
I looked in the mirror with unkind eyes, far too often.
I moved out of my first "big girl" apartment.
I ran the best roof deck in Newport, Rhode Island.
I can count on two hands the amount of times I purged (and I am so proud that I haven't purged since September).
I caught a lot of flights (and maybe a few feelings along the way).
I drank wine in Napa and a Hand Grenade at Mardi Gras.
I climbed a mountain in Bali, went to a tabernacle in Utah, and saw the Bean in Chicago.
I turned twenty-four!?!
I dyed my hair purple... like four times.
I said "see you later" to friends who turned into family and "goodbye" to friends who have become strangers.
I did some things I regret.
I celebrated love with my people who got engaged.
I couldn't tell you if I ate more oysters or dumplings.
I laughed loud and hugged tight.
I got one more tattoo and two more piercings.
I soaked in every single Rhode Island sunset.
I spend so much time feeling disconnected from myself.
I fought a losing battle and I'm still in the middle of it.
I'd be lying if I said I didn't want to start my year with a new gym membership and strict diet.
Truthfully, I ended the year feeling like a hot mess.

I don't really make resolutions. I've had the same one since I was nineteen years old: to continue to mend the relationship with myself and to try to make the most of every day.

With all of that being said, I want you to know that it's okay. It is okay to go into the new year struggling, I know I am. A change in date does not erase all of the pain you are carrying from the year before. But, if the new year proves anything, it's that whatever tried to beat you, lost.

I am so proud of you for making it to 2023. Happy New Year, angel.

Everyday can be January 1 if you have the right mindset.

2023
the year I filled the space that once scared me

Mirror, mirror, on the wall
Have I been this beautiful all along?

My body and skin do not compare
To the strength and kindness I always wear.

Mirror, mirror, on the wall
I was meant to be more than small.

My big, bold, and beautiful life
Is on the other side of all this strife

You damn mirror, on my wall
Why did I give you so much power, after all?

You only show a reflection that goes skin deep
And no matter what you see, my worth is for me to keep.

My dad always says, "Food is a time and a place."

I think that is really cool.

If you drink a glass of wine after you got the best news of your life, with your favorite person in the world, at a beautiful place, it will taste much different than if you drank it for the first time on a crummy day.

Maybe that is why I went to wine school, because each glass tells a story behind it. You don't need a hundred-dollar bottle or a steak dinner to experience this. A huge part of my healing was allowing myself to embrace myself in the combination of food and wine. And those combos can come from anywhere.

Cabernet Sauvignon, and Dark Chocolate (2016 Selah is my personal favorite)
Champagne and French Fries
Sauvignon Blanc, New Zealand and a Caesar Salad
Sancerre and a Cheese Board (don't forget the blue cheese and honey)
Prosecco and Chocolate Chip Pancakes
Riesling (dry or off-dry) and Sushi (with extra spicy mayo, of course)
Chianti and Meatballs
Rose Cava and Pork Roll, Egg and Cheese on a Jersey Bagel
Shiraz and anything drowned in BBQ sauce
Barolo and Burgers
Malbec and Goldfish
Pinot Noir, Oregon and Hummus
Rose and Hot Dogs (and a side of pasta salad)
Beaujolais and Turkey (on a sandwich or during Thanksgiving)

Peas in a pod.

2023

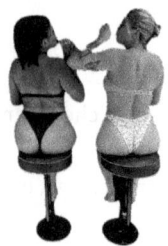

"We have to go here together,
let's plan a day"
- my longest friend, Neen

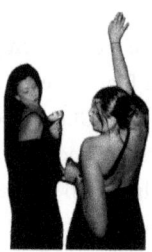

"I hope you are in my life forever."
- the girl I flew across the world
to find, Mar

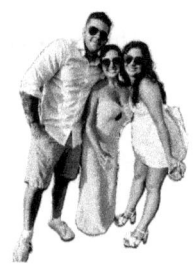

"Not a goodbye, just see you later."
- one big happy family

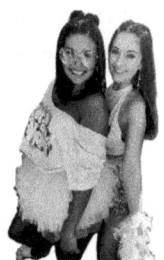

"Checking in!"
- we finish everything how we start it:
together, my Gianna

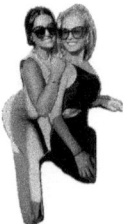

"You mean the world to me"
- my dearest roommate, Gwen

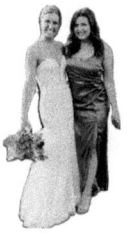

"I cannot wait to build OUR life together"
- the big sister I never had, Kel

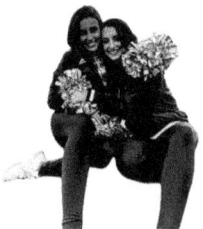

"Sweetest dreams!"
- my atom buddy, my seed, my forever friend, Serena

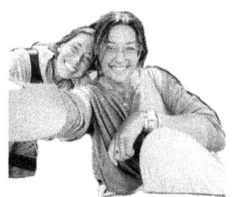

"224 (today, tomorrow, forever), 4444, worldwide!"
- my pen pal, Katie

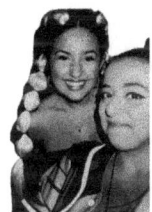

"I am so thankful for you."
- my sweet sweet Jamie

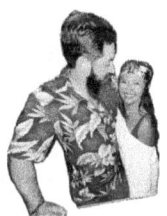

"The world needs more people like you."
- my pal Carl, #TeamTenn, #LWD

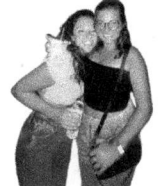

"Until our paths cross again!"
- my little bean, Ava

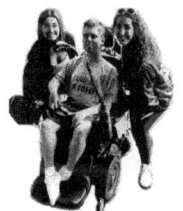

"I miss you."
- the strongest guy I know, Matt

Get yourself friends who say this

Songs to feel to.

Songs to feel (good) to.

I'll never forget when I was bartending, I had a woman say to me,

"I quit smoking two weeks ago and I really want a cigarette right now. What do I do?"

After pausing for a minute, I attempted to put myself in her shoes to sense what she needed in that moment. I tried to reason with her and remind her why she quit in the first place. I tried to help her realize she didn't want a physical cigarette, but wanted to feel the comfort and security smoking brought her. I ended by telling her she was stronger than her addiction and she will wake up tomorrow feeling so proud she didn't give in.

She left a little bit later, and that is where our story ends. I was just her bartender but I truly think about our interaction a lot. She took the first step. She found the strength to quit for two weeks. She asked a stranger for guidance when she needed it most. She's right there. All she needed to do was dig deep and hang in there.

I think we all could relate to her in some way: I know I've been there with my eating disorder.

Feeling there is something wrong with my body and the only way to fix it is leaning on my disordered behaviors.
Telling myself I have things under control and a few days of restricting won't hurt me.
Silently fighting the urge to slip back into my old ways and wishing someone would catch me and tell me not to.

So . . . to you,

I'm not sure what battle you are fighting: I've never walked in your shoes. I'm not sure what kind of week you are having: I don't know how your day has been or how you are feeling right now.

But what I do know is, whether today is the day you hit rock bottom or the day where everything "clicked"—I hear you and I am rooting for you.

Whether you decide to smoke your cigarette or not does not define you.

There are people out there in the world who care about you, many of them whom you haven't even met yet.
When you can't stay strong for yourself, do it for them. And more importantly, do it for your future self who is so proud of everything you are doing right now.

I don't know if she ever went on to find a cigarette that night. But what I do know, she will beat this and you will too.

We all have a cigarette we are unsure if we should light.

2023

I've always been the person to say, "I have so much love to give."

So, I filled my life with over-committing and overworking myself so I could impact as many people as possible.

Now I'm thinking, maybe the only person you need to make an impact on is yourself. Maybe that's when you make your greatest mark on the world.

Maybe you are your #1. Your best friend. Your hero after all.

Maybe just maybe, all that love that is inside of you should be shown to yourself, first.

Love yourself first.
Even if everyone else has, do not abandon you.

My pen pal, Katie, and I are cautious of our words. We are determined to change our narratives.

We don't have things to "work through," we have things to "break through."

Instead of saying, "How are you?" we ask, "How can I support you today?"

Rather than assuming what the other needs, we ask, "Do you need a distraction, a soundboard, or advice?"

She taught me how to set boundaries, show effort, and communicate effectively.

I have only seen her in person twice.

We have built the truest form of friendship, without seeing each other. If that doesn't prove that what you look like is the least interesting thing about you, I'm not sure what will.

2023

There are two types of people in this world: those who have been skydiving and those who haven't.

Some people jump to conquer their fears. Others jump for the adventure.

After I landed from the 15,000-foot free fall, I realized that jumping out of a plane in Hawaii wasn't going to free me from all of my fears. It wasn't going to release me of all anxiety I held onto before.

But it would remind me that I am capable of things that my mind can't comprehend.
That my "fear of heights" was a label that I put on something much deeper.

And if it reminded me of nothing else, it showed me that I am one heck of a badass.

Thank you for the visit in the sky, Dom.

I wonder what the boy who told me to "go for a run because I needed to lose some weight" would say about my bigger body.

I wonder what the person who told me "Saying 'normalize normal bodies' [a phrase written by Mik Zazon that changed my perspective when I needed it most] is an excuse to get fat" would think if they knew what really goes on behind the scenes.

I wonder what the woman who told me "We don't carry dresses in your size" would say to me now that I'm a size bigger.

I wonder what my first nutritionist who had me on a restrictive plan would say about my eating habits now.

As I wonder about all these things, I can't help but wonder what my life would be like if I never took the first step toward recovery.
If I never put myself first.
If I chose gym classes over lunch dates.
If I stopped dancing in the rain.
If I kept ordering gutted bagels and burgers without buns.
If I decided to be ashamed of my story, instead of sharing it.

I will always wonder if they knew what their words meant to me. I will always wonder what they would think of me now. With all of that wondering, I am so glad I will never have to wonder what my life would be like, if I still believed them.

The body I'm in allows me to:

Make it through a 14-hour shift on my feet.
Go to the gym on a random morning after not going for two months.
Take impulsive day trips anywhere and everywhere.
Say yes to dinner and drinks with my roommates.
It allows me to adventure as far as I can go, eat new things, and completely live in the moment.

The body that I'm in has supported me every single day.
It keeps going, even when I don't think it can.
It stays strong, even when all I do is try to beat it down.
It has my back, even when I turn mine on it.

The body that I'm in is the best gift I could've ever received. And even on my worst of days, I am so thankful for it.

Something to read over when your negative thoughts are raging loud.

You don't need to be published to be a writer.
You don't need a standing ovation to be a dancer.
You don't need a title to be a leader.
You don't need a specific BMI to be an athlete.
You don't need a cape to be a hero.

Stop selling yourself short.

2023

A full recovery is possible.

UNKNOWN WARRIOR

Everyone keeps asking me what I'm feeling. Nervous? Excited? Scared?

Right now, I'm feeling all the feels.

I'm remembering when I went to Rhode Island for the very first time and I wailed in my mom's arms because I was so afraid to go. (And going there changed my life for the better.)

I'm remembering when I ate an incredible meal at this exact restaurant and purged it all. (And looking back at it, I just wanna give that girl on the bathroom floor a hug.)

I remember a younger me who dreamed of seeing the world and an older me who just wanted to leave her mark on it.

And I'm doing just that.

I'm having my send-off dinner at the restaurant I've felt my lowest. I looked in the mirror as I was getting ready and saw the girl who was too afraid to cross the road, let alone the ocean.

I'm feeling happy, a little sad, but most of all, I'm feeling proud of the woman I've become. I am honored to be moving across the world tomorrow to be a mentor to kids who don't have one.

Let's save the world.

Ciao!

The night before I started one of my greatest adventures.
Stop #2 of my Eat, Pray, Love journey.

I was drawn to Italy. So, I packed my bags, hopped on a flight, and moved to Rome for three months to volunteer in the hopes of finding a home within myself, across the world.

I discovered blood orange Powerade.
I took the escalator instead of the stairs.
I realized I was a great teacher.
I (mentally) ended a 10-plus-year love affair I held onto in my head.
I tried a new red wine.
I got a liter of white wine for 4 euros at the supermarket.
I skipped breakfast.
I met Mar, Sharon, Aurora, Isabelle, Paula, Isa, Kat, Naomi, Ann, Becca, and Xanthe.
I got a hug from one of the kids I am mentoring.
I got a kiss on both cheeks from my supervisor.
I texted all of my people to let me know when they woke up on the 16th [a poignant date when I lost someone close to me].
I kinda miss New Jersey.
I really miss my family.
I need to keep my head on straight.
I gotta stay strong.
I tried my first cappuccino.
I ate black truffles and gelato.
I went to a rooftop.
I looked at myself with kind eyes.
I am doing it.

I sang "Special" by Lizzo on stage at a packed Irish Pub on karaoke night. I may have (and by may have I mean I absolutely) said, "You are more than your body, and what you look like is the least interesting thing about you."
I taught an ESL class to a room full of Italians—who spoke zero English—and mentioned that Americans put pineapple on pizza ... it did not go over well.

And it's only day 5 of 90 in Rome. My love cup is overflowing.

I made it one week here without craving sushi. A few girls and I went to a surprisingly great Japanese restaurant. Our server told us that there was only one chef and that our food was going to take a little while. We didn't mind, we were just happy to be there. He brought us edamame for us to enjoy.

A few moments later he comes back and says, "These are from the kitchen as well."

... yes, you guessed it. DUMPLINGS.

I swear I shed a tear. I know this Japanese restaurant will be one of my favorite Italian memories.

Dumplings 2.0
This was definitely a "Sunset" page.

2023

Food neutrality in Italy is un-freaking-real.

There is no such thing as good or bad. The pasta section on the menu is always the largest one. There is no "dieter's choice" page. There are never any calories listed.

You stop and sit at a café for a cappuccino at any point in the day, and stay as long as you like. You casually eat gelato no matter what time it is. To say it is life-changing and eye-opening is the definition of an understatement.

Getting my #CALLAries in throughout Italy.
I love this country.

Could you imagine how utterly ridiculous it would be if we labeled other things as good or bad like we do food?

Good pillows
Bad plates
Good doorknobs
Bad ceiling fans
Good remote controls
Bad cabinets

2023

While asking our taxi driver what we should fill our seventy-two hours in Ireland with, he replied (in his thick Irish accent),

"Don't sleep in. Don't sleep past breakfast. Unless you have a hot blarney with you. Let them stay as long as they like."

He then went on to say, on a more serious note,

"There is always something to miss. Don't spend 10 hours doing 50 things. Spend 10 hours doing 10 things and enjoy all of them to the fullest. You want to go to the wax museum? Do it. It's f*cking stupid. But if you don't go, you're missing it. There's a bar next to it. It's crap, but if you don't go, you're missing it. You'll always miss something, *so don't miss the places you actually go.*"

And I thought that was kinda beautiful.

When in ~~Rome~~ Ireland . . .

I got into another taxi with my suitcase when I returned to Rome.

As my driver went to put it in his trunk I said, "Sorry it's so heavy!"

He looked at me and deadass replied, "A heavy bag for a heavy girl."

Ohhhhhh Mr. Sir, before you go f yourself, I encourage you to take a good long look at me and see:

My big heart.
My big personality.
My big dreams.
My big ole back side.
My strong legs.
My strong curves.
My strong mind.
My strong sense of self.

After you notice all of that, maybe then I won't mind being called heavy, because your words reflect you a hell of a lot more than they will ever reflect me.

I will forever be confused as to why people feel the need to make unsolicited, uneducated, and uncalled-for comments about my body. But I will forever be thankful for the big, strong, beautiful body I'm in.

If only my Irish driver came back to Italy with me.

2023

I was having one of the worst body image days I've experienced since being in Italy. My mind kept echoing the cruel mantra: *Since you're one of the "larger girls" here, you have to make up for it in other ways.*

I slipped back into my old habit of trying to compensate in other ways—anything to divert attention from my size.

I felt like I was trapped in a dark place, struggling with every step. Reluctantly, I headed to dinner. As we passed a crepe shop on our way to the bar, I hesitated but followed inside. There, I saw a sign that struck a chord with me:

*"F*ck the diet."*

It was the reminder I needed.

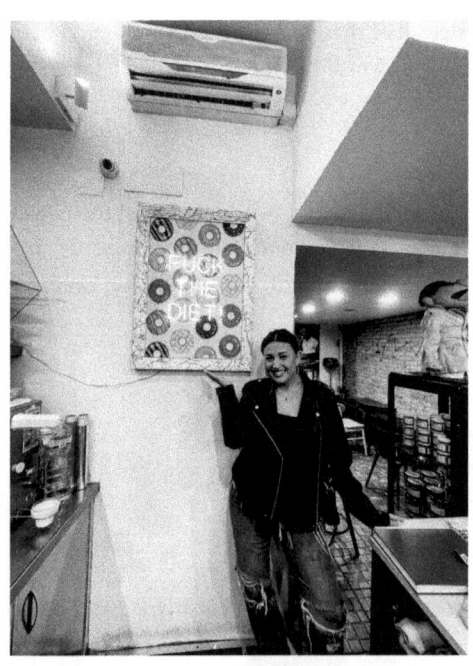

I learned sign language so I could better communicate with one of the new volunteers at my placement.

I talked to the guy who owned the minimart next to the bus stop (where I would go every single day and get a blood orange Powerade) so we could get to know each other.

I befriended everyone who worked at my favorite Irish pub so they felt like humans instead of vending machines.

I see these people all of the time. They could be people in the background. But everyone has a story and I wanted to know theirs.

Eight billion people in the world, and every single one can impact your life.

All you have to do is let them.

I wish I could tell younger me being wheeled into surgery that she hasn't met all of the people who are going to love her yet.

2023

I am late for everything.

Zoom meetings.
Breakfast plans.
Flights.
Doctor's appointments.

Yeah, that's it.
This is the page.
No deeper meaning, this is just how I live my life. Oops.

This would've been a "Somewhere around 2 a.m." page.

Last book break!!!!

Have you fueled your body today?

If you haven't yet, please go do so.

Your body and I thank you.

2023

I give people grace for using me as a topic of conversations I'm not a part of.

- I went random and met my roommate, Gwen, on move-in day.
- I offered to drive my teammate, Serena, home from practice.
- I called a new friend, Katie, on a long drive home.
- I chose Rhode Island.
- I accepted the Roof Deck job promotion.
- I scheduled an appointment with [who is now] my current therapist, Jenny.
- I booked a flight to Bali.
- I signed up to volunteer in Italy.
- I used the buddy system on my first night there with Mar.

Every single one of these moments seemed insignificant at the time and they changed my life forever.

My reason to believe everything happens for a reason.
All it takes is twenty seconds of instant courage, right?

2023

I have lived as a stranger in my body.
For so long, I let time pass me by.
I put so much effort into making a living and a name for myself that I forgot to make myself a life.
I was so focused on not dropping the weight of the world, I didn't let myself see all the people there to help me carry it.
I was always bracing for impact so when joy was around me, I never truly let it in.

It's time to find you again. It's time to go back home to yourself.

I went to dinner with an old friend, Gianna, at an all-you-can-eat sushi restaurant after not seeing each other for years. We didn't look at the menu for the healthiest option. We talked like no time passed at all and had the best sushi ever. It was awesome.

I went to lunch with my friend's friends. I don't think I talked a lot—I was too consumed by their stories. I had never felt so whole. I was taken out of my bubble and let myself feel the love they had for each other. It was the most incredible feeling.

I went to a bar in Bali and got drinks with girls I had only met a few days prior. We all traveled solo and found people that made across the world feel at home. We asked the DJ if we could play our music and had a dance party in the pool that was in the middle of the restaurant. It will always be one of my favorite memories.

I went to the bus station in Italy and as we were waiting to get on, I told my friends, "I heard you need four hugs a day for a good quality of life." We all went in a circle, gave each other tight hugs, and then adventured until the sun went down. It was beautiful.

I went to work one day and someone from a leadership camp I met eight years ago—for only four days—messaged me that they were in Rhode Island. They came to visit and we talked like old friends, when on paper we were more like strangers. It was such a grounding moment.

You never know who you impact.
There are more people who care about you than you will ever know.

Connections that defy time and distance.

2023

Did you catch the news this morning?

I heard it is projected to be the best day ever.

The very first thing I say every day when I walk into work.

When I journal, I imagine myself standing there.

But not me in that moment. I don't picture a specific outfit. I don't see my cellulite or body rolls. I don't see my accolades or job title.

For a split second, I see my soul. I see my true self.

And that girl is smiling with tears in her eyes. She is the strongest girl I know. She has some broken pieces, but she will be damned before she lets someone tell her she's broken.

She needs a hug. She is tired. Sometimes, it feels like she's hanging on by a thread.

When I journal, it isn't so easy to tear myself apart. All the insults and negative thoughts don't come so easily. I don't even let other people in my mind to compare myself to.

They say it is hard to hate others up close. Maybe that is because you see people for who they truly are.

Next time you put pen to paper, give this mentality a try.

Now that I'm here, I realize I haven't cried in a long time. I guess I'm crying because of it all. I can't believe I'm writing this book. I can't believe I moved back to Rhode Island. I can't believe I haven't met all the people who are going to love me. I also can't believe I have hurt so deeply for so long. I can't believe this world has lost some people way too soon. I just really can't wrap my head around everything right now, so I am just going to sit here and cry until I have no tears left and wake up tomorrow and just believe today is a new day.

A voice message I left for myself.

I can't believe I'm still standing.
The "Storm" page.

Why are all my friends so far away?
Why is everything so expensive?
Why can't I drive to Italy?
Why can't you apply for a job to change the world?

I know your twenties are supposed to be a mess, but what the f*ck?
I still don't have all the answers,
but I will always be someone who has been there.

Some people dream about their bank account having a certain number of zeroes.

Other people dream about the moment they have that car, that job, or that partner.

For me, I dream about the day I look in the mirror and, with only my reflection staring back at me, say... "I'm home."

One day soon.

I think I'm so tired all the time because my broken pieces are heavy and there are a lot of them to pick up and it is something I have had to do every day . . .

. . . by myself

. . . and make it look effortless

I asked the people closest to me to send me their favorite memories of us. Some of them included:

- Showing up to our guy friend's house in party hats and convincing them all we should have a celebratory Saturday for no reason.
- It was just two of us on New Year's and we didn't leave the couch or each other's side for four days.
- Hysterical laughing about her getting a 0 on her chem final.
- Trying to play True American (thank you, *New Girl*).
- Talking in our driveways for hours after getting home because we couldn't stop talking.
- When I texted her on our first day of UDA camp.
- Eating McFlurrys at the Sea Wall.

All these moments were just regular days. In the past years, my friends and I have traveled and accomplished so many things. But when it comes down to it, their favorite moments are the authentic and effortless ones.

I think that's really beautiful.

Don't let a glamorized ideation convince you otherwise.

UNKNOWN WARRIOR

The smaller size wasn't worth it.

You are what you cannot see.

Their battlefield was the dinner table.

Despite it all, they saved themselves.

Six-word stories.

I give super-tight hugs.
I eat dumplings whenever my big heart desires.
I sleep and sleep and sleep some more.
I wear clothes that accentuate my curves, not hide them.
I travel as far and as often as I can.
I find ways to move my body that aren't always at the gym.
I take up space and remind myself that it's okay to do so.
I dance around my kitchen all by myself.
I hold my head high.

I celebrate myself in the little moments . . .

. . . and it was the turning point in my healing journey.

UNKNOWN WARRIOR

Donate your hair.
Donate clothes you don't wear anymore.
Donate your time.
Donate a dollar. Donate five.

Speak up for those who are afraid.
Speak up for those who physically can't.
Speak up for those who are silenced.
Speak up for those things that matter.

Volunteer somewhere.
Host a bingo night at a nursing home.
Write letters to your local hospital.
Clean up the beach.
Write a good review for a small business.
Buy the person's coffee behind you.
Hold the door open for strangers.
Smile at someone.

Leave this world better than you found it.

2023

What made you happiest until you let the world alter you?

Journal Prompt 7.0

YOU ARE ONE BAD BITCH. DON'T LET ANYONE TELL YOU OTHERWISE.

It makes me so f*cking sad that you think it is better to starve yourself or to purge than to fuel your body.

You deserve so much more than this. You can't change the world on an empty stomach. And even though it is the least interesting thing about you, you are absolutely breathtaking just the way you are.

You are beautiful.

Don't just read over it.

Did you hear me?

Yes, you.

Let it sink in.
You are beautiful.

You
Are
Beautiful
You are beautiful for everything you are and everything you are not.

I hope you see that one day soon.

English

Mi rende così fottutamente triste che tu pensi che sia meglio morire di fame o epurazione piuttosto che alimentare il tuo corpo.

Ti meriti molto di più di questo. Non puoi cambiare il mondo a stomaco vuoto. E, anche se è la cosa meno interessante di te, sei assolutamente mozzafiato così come sei.

Sei bello.

Non limitarti a leggerlo.

Mi hai sentito?

Si tu.

Lascia che si consolidi.
Sei bello.

Voi
Sono
Bellissimo
Sei bella per tutto ciò che sei e per tutto ciò che non sei.

Spero che tu lo veda presto un giorno.

Italian

2023

2023 was nothing I thought it would be and everything I could've wished for.

I moved to Italy for three months.
Throughout those three months, I smiled bigger and learned more about myself than I ever thought possible.
I got four more tattoos.
I rekindled old friendships and made new ones . . . both of which I can only hope will last a lifetime.
I went skydiving in Hawaii.
I ate a TON of sushi.
I started my public speaking career with Greek University.
My weight fluctuated a lot.
I watched the entire series of *Law & Order: SVU* and now I live my life by asking myself, "What would Olivia Benson do?"
I drank a ridiculous amount of blue Powerade.
I went to my best friend's wedding alone and realized I am the best date I could ever ask for.
I purged . . . more than I'm proud of.
I tried to make Tennessee Avenue the best it could be.
I took off my eyelash extensions.
I cheered my sister on during her first show.
I found my favorite cocktail and second family at Little Water Distillery.
I made mistakes.
I got new acne scars.
I touched someone's life.
I officiated a stranger's wedding.
I met my nutritionist for the first time in person.
I broke down and cried, but I smiled and loved even more.

Not knowing what tomorrow will bring used to be something I feared, but no, it is something I look forward to. This year, I let go of wishing for a crystal ball and embraced the belief that the best is yet to come. Here's to 2024 being the best year yet.

Dear me,

I just wanted to say that I'm sorry.
I am sorry to the younger you, who was naive and gullible in believing she wasn't good enough.
I am sorry I wasn't there to hold you in your dark nights of anxiety-ridden thoughts.
I am sorry I was not strong enough to feed you when you needed it most.
I am sorry I abandoned you on the bathroom floor.
I am sorry I used my hand to purge rather than to hold yours to help you up.
I am sorry I looked at you with unkind eyes for so many years.
I am sorry for all of the times I turned my back on you.
I am sorry I was too stubborn to realize how incredible you are.
I am sorry I tried to shrink you; you were made for so much more than that.

More than anything, I am sorry it took me until now to say all of this to you.
Now . . .
You can breathe.
You can put it down.
You do not need to carry this by yourself anymore.

I am here with you. I am never leaving.
I forgive you.
I love you and I'm proud of you.

Xo,
Me

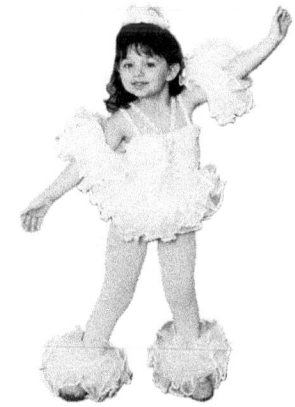

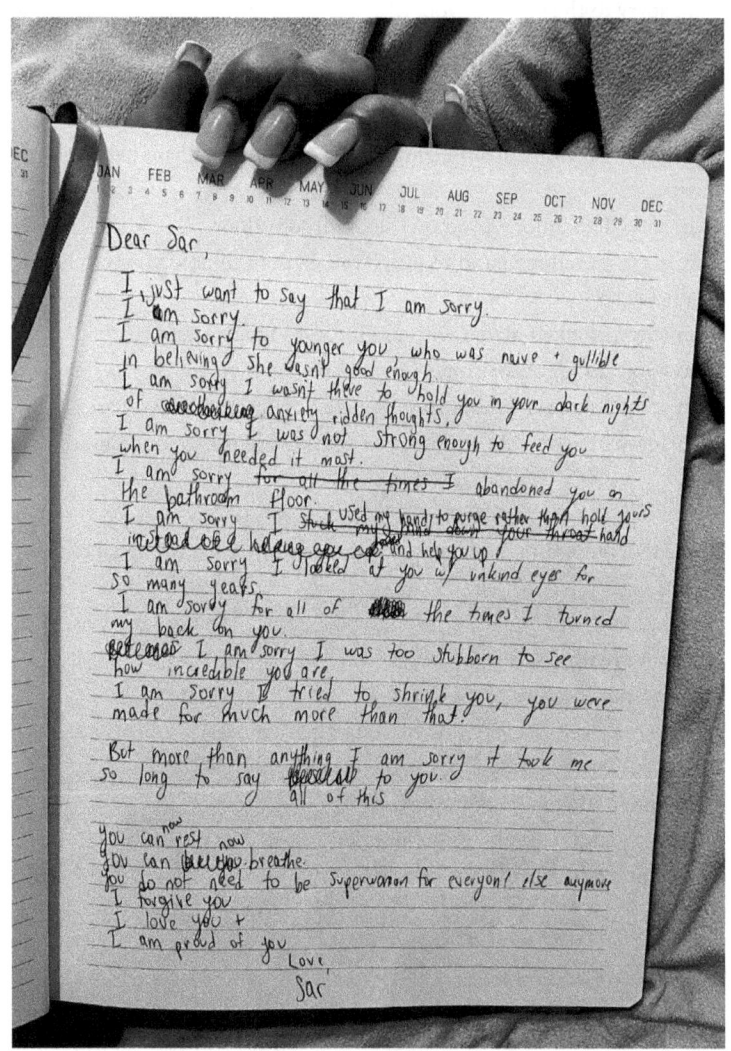

2024
the year that has only begun

Now it's time for me to pass the baton to you.

It's time for you to write a letter to yourself—whatever kind of letter you need. You can read it to someone close to you, burn it, or maybe end up publishing it one day.

It's time for you to look at yourself with kind eyes and show that little voice in your head that you are ready to fight.

It's time for you to close this book, go out into the world, and conquer all that life throws at you.

Hold your head high and know I am always a page away.

From the bottom of my heart, thank you for being here and for being you.
With every ounce of love in me,

Xo

Sar

Journal Prompt 8.0

For Further Resources

For more ways to support someone struggling with an eating disorder and get connected to resources . . .

Please scan below to message Sar.

Acknowledgments

I am deeply honored to acknowledge Greek University and its remarkable community. To be part of such an extraordinary group of powerhouse individuals is a privilege I will always treasure. Your unwavering belief in me, even when I struggled to believe in myself, has been a source of immense strength and inspiration.

A heartfelt thank-you goes out to Michael Ayalon and all my Greek U family members. Your support, encouragement, and genuine camaraderie have been invaluable to me throughout this journey. Your belief in my vision has helped me grow in ways I could never have imagined. Also, thank you to my editor, Amanda Varian.

For those inspired to collaborate with me or connect with any of my incredible friends, please visit https://greekuniversity.org/sarah/.

I would also like to take a moment to *not* acknowledge artificial intelligence. This book was crafted from the heart, without the aid of AI. I am proud to have created this work entirely by myself, for myself.

Dreams do come true. Thank you for being a part of my journey.
xo
Sar

About the Author

I am a proud University of Rhode Island alumni. After graduation, I quit what I thought was my dream marketing job and listened to my gut. Instead of following what I "should be doing," I am taking my twenties to live intuitively, making each day as big and bold as possible. I have been actively working on my eating disorder recovery for five years and in May of 2025 I will be graduating from Fairleigh Dickinson University with my Masters of Social Work.

I freaking love dumplings and feta cheese. I have nine tattoos. I am always late posting on BeReal. I have my Level 2 Sommelier certification and am a sushi/spicy mayo enthusiast. My camera roll is filled with pictures of my people and the world around us. I put my all into everything I do. I am an author, professional speaker, and advocate. I am struggling; I am strong.

Some things haven't changed. I still love watching Food Network like I did when I was a little girl. I'd still do anything for the people I care about. I am still learning to love myself.

Today and every day from here on out, I am choosing to be the person I want to be. And I hope you like her, because I'm really starting to.

www.ingramcontent.com/pod-product-compliance
Lightning Source LLC
Chambersburg PA
CBHW070623030426
42337CB00020B/3892